This report contains the collective views of an international group of experts and does not necessarily represent the decisions or the stated policy of the United Nations Environment Programme, the International Labour Organisation, or the World Health Organization.

Environmental Health Criteria 203

CHRYSOTILE ASBESTOS

First draft prepared by Dr G. Gibbs, Canada (Chapter 2), Mr B.J. Pigg, USA (Chapter 3), Professor W.J. Nicholson, USA (Chapter 4), Dr A. Morgan, UK and Professor M. Lippmann, USA (Chapter 5), Dr J.M.G. Davis, UK and Professor B.T. Mossman, USA (Chapter 6), Professor J.C. McDonald, UK, Professor P.J. Landrigan, USA and Professor W.J. Nicholson, USA (Chapter 7), Professor H. Schreier, Canada (Chapter 8).

Published under the joint sponsorship of the United Nations Environment Programme, the International Labour Organisation, and the World Health Organization, and produced within the framework of the Inter-Organization Programme for the Sound Management of Chemicals.

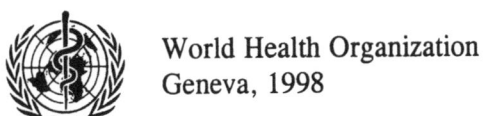

World Health Organization
Geneva, 1998

The **International Programme on Chemical Safety (IPCS)**, established in 1980, is a joint venture of the United Nations Environment Programme (UNEP), the International Labour Organisation (ILO), and the World Health Organization (WHO). The overall objectives of the IPCS are to establish the scientific basis for assessment of the risk to human health and the environment from exposure to chemicals, through international peer review processes, as a prerequisite for the promotion of chemical safety, and to provide technical assistance in strengthening national capacities for the sound management of chemicals.

The **Inter-Organization Programme for the Sound Management of Chemicals (IOMC)** was established in 1995 by UNEP, ILO, the Food and Agriculture Organization of the United Nations, WHO, the United Nations Industrial Development Organization, the United Nations Institute for Training and Research, and the Organisation for Economic Co-operation and Development (Participating Organizations), following recommendations made by the 1992 UN Conference on Environment and Development to strengthen cooperation and increase coordination in the field of chemical safety. The purpose of the IOMC is to promote coordination of the policies and activities pursued by the Participating Organizations, jointly or separately, to achieve the sound management of chemicals in relation to human health and the environment.

WHO Library Cataloguing in Publication Data

Chrysotile Asbestos.

(Environmental health criteria ; 203)

1.Asbestos, Serpentine - adverse effects 2.Asbestos, Serpentine - toxicity
3.Environmental exposure 4.Occupational exposure I.International Programme on Chemical Safety II.Series

ISBN 92 4 157203 5   (NLM Classification: WA 754)
ISSN 0250-863X

The World Health Organization welcomes requests for permission to reproduce or translate its publications, in part or in full. Applications and enquiries should be addressed to the Office of Publications, World Health Organization, Geneva, Switzerland, which will be glad to provide the latest information on any changes made to the text, plans for new editions, and reprints and translations already available.

©World Health Organization 1998

Publications of the World Health Organization enjoy copyright protection in accordance with the provisions of Protocol 2 of the Universal Copyright Convention. All rights reserved.

The designations employed and the presentation of the material in this publication do not imply the expression of any opinion whatsoever on the part of the Secretariat of the World Health Organization concerning the legal status of any country, territory, city, or area or of its authorities, or concerning the delimitation of its frontiers or boundaries.

The mention of specific companies or of certain manufacturers' products does not imply that they are endorsed or recommended by the World Health Organization in preference to others of a similar nature that are not mentioned. Errors and omissions excepted, the names of proprietary products are distinguished by initial capital letters.

PRINTED IN FINLAND
98/12141 – VAMMALA – 5000

CONTENTS

ENVIRONMENTAL HEALTH CRITERIA FOR CHRYSOTILE ASBESTOS

PREAMBLE	ix
ABBREVIATIONS	xix
INTRODUCTION	xx
1. SUMMARY	1
1.1 Identity, physical and chemical properties, sampling and analysis	1
1.2 Sources of occupational and environmental exposure	2
1.3 Occupational and environmental exposure levels	2
1.4 Uptake, clearance, retention and translocation	4
1.5 Effects on animals and cells	5
1.6 Effects on humans	7
1.7 Environmental fate and effects on biota	9
2. IDENTITY, PHYSICAL AND CHEMICAL PROPERTIES, SAMPLING AND ANALYSIS	10
2.1 Identity	10
2.1.1 Chemical composition	10
2.1.2 Structure	10
2.1.3 Fibre forms in the ore	11
2.1.4 Fibre properties	11
2.1.5 UICC samples	12
2.1.6 Associated minerals in chrysotile ore	12
2.2 Physical and chemical properties	14
2.2.1 Physical properties	14
2.2.2 Chemical properties	16
2.3 Sampling and analytical methods	16
2.3.1 Workplace sampling	17
2.3.2 Sampling in the general environment	17

	2.3.3	Analytical methods	18
		2.3.3.1 Fibre identification	18
		2.3.3.2 Measurement of airborne fibre concentrations	19
		2.3.3.3 Lung tissue analysis	20
		2.3.3.4 Gravimetric analysis	20
2.4	Conversion factors		20
	2.4.1	Conversion from airborne particle to fibre concentrations	21
	2.4.2	Conversion from total mass to fibre number concentrations	22

3. SOURCES OF OCCUPATIONAL AND ENVIRONMENTAL EXPOSURE   23

    3.1 Natural occurrence   23
    3.2 Anthropogenic sources   23
        3.2.1 Production   24
        3.2.2 Manufacture of products   27
        3.2.3 Use of products   28

4. OCCUPATIONAL AND ENVIRONMENTAL EXPOSURE LEVELS   30

    4.1 Occupational exposure   30
        4.1.1 Mining and milling   31
        4.1.2 Textile production   33
        4.1.3 Asbestos-cement   39
        4.1.4 Friction products   40
        4.1.5 Exposure of building maintenance personnel   41
        4.1.6 Various industries   45
    4.2 Non-occupational exposure   47
        4.2.1 Ambient air   47
        4.2.2 Indoor air   47

5. UPTAKE, CLEARANCE, RETENTION AND TRANSLOCATION   51

		5.1	Inhalation			51
			5.1.1	General principles		51
			5.1.2	Fibre deposition		54
			5.1.3	Fibre clearance and retention		55
				5.1.3.1	Fibre clearance and retention in humans	55
				5.1.3.2	Fibre clearance and retention in laboratory animals	55
			5.1.4	Fibre translocation		64
				5.1.4.1	Fibre translocation in humans	64
				5.1.4.2	Fibre translocation in animal models	65
			5.1.5	Mechanisms of fibre clearance		66
		5.2	Ingestion			68
6.	EFFECTS ON LABORATORY MAMMALS AND *IN VITRO* TEST SYSTEMS					69
		6.1	Introduction			69
		6.2	Effects on laboratory mammals			70
			6.2.1	Summary of previous studies		70
			6.2.2	Recent long-term inhalation studies		71
			6.2.3	Intratracheal and intrabronchial injection studies		78
			6.2.4	Intraperitoneal and intrapleural injection studies		81
			6.2.5	Ingestion studies		91
		6.3	Studies on cells			93
			6.3.1	Genotoxicity and interactions with DNA		93
			6.3.2	Cell proliferation		97
			6.3.3	Inflammation		99
			6.3.4	Cell death and cytotoxicity		100
			6.3.5	Liberation of growth factors and other response of cells of the immune system		101
7.	EFFECTS ON HUMANS					103
		7.1	Occupational exposure			103

	7.1.1	Pneumoconiosis and other non-malignant respiratory effects	103
	7.1.2	Lung cancer and mesothelioma	106
		7.1.2.1 Critical occupational cohort studies – chrysotile	107
		7.1.2.2 Comparisons of lung cancer exposure-response – critical studies	118
		7.1.2.3 Other relevant studies	120
	7.1.3	Other malignant diseases	125
		7.1.3.1 Critical occupational cohort studies involving chrysotile	126
		7.1.3.2 Other relevant studies	127
7.2	Non-occupational exposure		127

8. ENVIRONMENTAL FATE AND EFFECTS ON BIOTA 129

    8.1   Environmental transport and distribution   129
         8.1.1   Chrysotile fibres in water   129
         8.1.2   Chrysotile fibres in soil   130
    8.2   Effects on biota   130
         8.2.1   Impact on plants   131
         8.2.2   Impact on terrestrial life-forms   132
         8.2.3   Impact on aquatic biota   133

9. EVALUATION OF HEALTH RISKS OF EXPOSURE TO CHRYSOTILE ASBESTOS 136

    9.1   Introduction   136
    9.2   Exposure   137
         9.2.1   Occupational exposure   137
                9.2.1.1   Production   137
                9.2.1.2   Use   138
         9.2.2   General population exposure   139
    9.3   Health effects   140
         9.3.1   Occupational exposure   140
                9.3.1.1   Fibrosis   141
                9.3.1.2   Lung cancer   142

		9.3.1.3 Mesothelioma	142
	9.3.2	General environment	143
9.4	Effects on the environment		143

10. CONCLUSIONS AND RECOMMENDATIONS FOR PROTECTION OF HUMAN HEALTH — 144

11. FURTHER RESEARCH — 145

REFERENCES — 146

RÉSUMÉ — 176

RESUMEN — 187

NOTE TO READERS OF THE CRITERIA MONOGRAPHS

Every effort has been made to present information in the criteria monographs as accurately as possible without unduly delaying their publication. In the interest of all users of the Environmental Health Criteria monographs, readers are requested to communicate any errors that may have occurred to the Director of the International Programme on Chemical Safety, World Health Organization, Geneva, Switzerland, in order that they may be included in corrigenda.

* * *

A detailed data profile and a legal file can be obtained from the International Register of Potentially Toxic Chemicals, Case postale 356, 1219 Châtelaine, Geneva, Switzerland (telephone no. + 41 22 – 9799111, fax no. + 41 22 – 7973460, E-mail irptc@unep.ch).

* * *

This publication was made possible by grant number 5 U01 ES02617-15 from the National Institute of Environmental Health Sciences, National Institutes of Health, USA, and by financial support from the European Commission.

Environmental Health Criteria

PREAMBLE

Objectives

In 1973 the WHO Environmental Health Criteria Programme was initiated with the following objectives:

(i) to assess information on the relationship between exposure to environmental pollutants and human health, and to provide guidelines for setting exposure limits;

(ii) to identify new or potential pollutants;

(iii) to identify gaps in knowledge concerning the health effects of pollutants;

(iv) to promote the harmonization of toxicological and epidemiological methods in order to have internationally comparable results.

The first Environmental Health Criteria (EHC) monograph, on mercury, was published in 1976 and since that time an ever-increasing number of assessments of chemicals and of physical effects have been produced. In addition, many EHC monographs have been devoted to evaluating toxicological methodology, e.g., for genetic, neurotoxic, teratogenic and nephrotoxic effects. Other publications have been concerned with epidemiological guidelines, evaluation of short-term tests for carcinogens, biomarkers, effects on the elderly and so forth.

Since its inauguration the EHC Programme has widened its scope, and the importance of environmental effects, in addition to health effects, has been increasingly emphasized in the total evaluation of chemicals.

The original impetus for the Programme came from World Health Assembly resolutions and the recommendations of the 1972 UN Conference on the Human Environment. Subsequently the work became an integral part of the International Programme on Chemical Safety (IPCS), a cooperative programme of UNEP, ILO and WHO. In this manner, with the strong support of the new partners, the importance of occupational health and environmental effects was fully recognized. The EHC monographs have become widely established, used and recognized throughout the world.

The recommendations of the 1992 UN Conference on Environment and Development and the subsequent establishment of the Intergovernmental Forum on Chemical Safety with the priorities for action in the six programme areas of Chapter 19, Agenda 21, all lend further weight to the need for EHC assessments of the risks of chemicals.

Scope

The criteria monographs are intended to provide critical reviews on the effect on human health and the environment of chemicals and of combinations of chemicals and physical and biological agents. As such, they include and review studies that are of direct relevance for the evaluation. However, they do not describe *every* study carried out. Worldwide data are used and are quoted from original studies, not from abstracts or reviews. Both published and unpublished reports are considered and it is incumbent on the authors to assess all the articles cited in the references. Preference is always given to published data. Unpublished data are only used when relevant published data are absent or when they are pivotal to the risk assessment. A detailed policy statement is available that describes the procedures used for unpublished proprietary data so that this information can be used in the evaluation without compromising its confidential nature (WHO (1990) Revised Guidelines for the Preparation of Environmental Health Criteria Monographs. PCS/90.69, Geneva, World Health Organization).

In the evaluation of human health risks, sound human data, whenever available, are preferred to animal data. Animal and *in vitro* studies provide support and are used mainly to supply evidence missing from human studies. It is mandatory that research on human subjects is conducted in full accord with ethical principles, including the provisions of the Helsinki Declaration.

The EHC monographs are intended to assist national and international authorities in making risk assessments and subsequent risk management decisions. They represent a thorough evaluation of risks and are not, in any sense, recommendations for regulation or standard setting. These latter are the exclusive purview of national and regional governments.

Content

The layout of EHC monographs for chemicals is outlined below.

- Summary — a review of the salient facts and the risk evaluation of the chemical
- Identity — physical and chemical properties, analytical methods
- Sources of exposure
- Environmental transport, distribution and transformation
- Environmental levels and human exposure
- Kinetics and metabolism in laboratory animals and humans
- Effects on laboratory mammals and *in vitro* test systems
- Effects on humans
- Effects on other organisms in the laboratory and field
- Evaluation of human health risks and effects on the environment
- Conclusions and recommendations for protection of human health and the environment
- Further research
- Previous evaluations by international bodies, e.g., IARC, JECFA, JMPR

Selection of chemicals

Since the inception of the EHC Programme, the IPCS has organized meetings of scientists to establish lists of priority chemicals for subsequent evaluation. Such meetings have been held in: Ispra, Italy, 1980; Oxford, United Kingdom, 1984; Berlin, Germany, 1987; and North Carolina, USA, 1995. The selection of chemicals has been based on the following criteria: the existence of scientific evidence that the substance presents a hazard to human health and/or the environment; the possible use, persistence, accumulation or degradation of the substance shows that there may be significant human or environmental exposure; the size and nature of populations at risk (both human and other species) and risks for environment; international concern, i.e. the substance is of major interest to several countries; adequate data on the hazards are available.

If an EHC monograph is proposed for a chemical not on the priority list, the IPCS Secretariat consults with the Cooperating Organizations and all the Participating Institutions before embarking on the preparation of the monograph.

Procedures

The order of procedures that result in the publication of an EHC monograph is shown in the flow chart. A designated staff member of IPCS, responsible for the scientific quality of the document, serves as Responsible Officer (RO). The IPCS Editor is responsible for layout and language. The first draft, prepared by consultants or, more usually, staff from an IPCS Participating Institution, is based initially on data provided from the International Register of Potentially Toxic Chemicals, and reference data bases such as Medline and Toxline.

The draft document, when received by the RO, may require an initial review by a small panel of experts to determine its scientific quality and objectivity. Once the RO finds the document acceptable as a first draft, it is distributed, in its unedited form, to well over 150 EHC contact points throughout the world who are asked to comment on its completeness and accuracy and, where necessary, provide additional material. The contact points, usually designated by governments, may be Participating Institutions, IPCS Focal Points, or individual scientists known for their particular expertise. Generally some four months are allowed before the comments are considered by the RO and author(s). A second draft incorporating comments received and approved by the Director, IPCS, is then distributed to Task Group members, who carry out the peer review, at least six weeks before their meeting.

The Task Group members serve as individual scientists, not as representatives of any organization, government or industry. Their function is to evaluate the accuracy, significance and relevance of the information in the document and to assess the health and environmental risks from exposure to the chemical. A summary and recommendations for further research and improved safety aspects are also required. The composition of the Task Group is dictated by the range of expertise required for the subject of the meeting and by the need for a balanced geographical distribution.

EHC PREPARATION FLOW CHART

```
                    ┌─────────────────────────┐
                    │ Commitment to draft EHC │
                    └───────────┬─────────────┘
                                ▼
                    ┌─────────────────────────┐
           ┌ ─ ─ ─ ─│ Document preparation    │─ ─ ─ ─ ┐
           │        │ initiated               │        │
           │        └───────────┬─────────────┘        │
           ▼                    ▼                      ▼
┌──────────────┐   ┌─────────────────────────┐   ┌────────────────┐
│ Revision as  │◄──│ Draft sent to IPCS      │◄──│ Possible meeting│
│ necessary    │   │ Responsible Officer (RO)│   │ of a few experts│
└──────────────┘   └───────────┬─────────────┘   │ to resolve      │
                               ▼                 │ controversial   │
                   ┌─────────────────────────────┐ │ issues        │
                   │ Responsible Officer, Editor │ └────────────────┘
                   │ check for coherence of text │
                   │ and readability (not        │
                   │ language editing)           │
                   └───────────┬─────────────────┘
                               ▼
                    ┌─────────────────────────┐
                    │      First Draft        │
                    └───────────┬─────────────┘
                                ▼
                   ┌──────────────────────────────┐
                   │ International circulation to │
                   │ Contact Points (150+)        │
                   └───────────┬──────────────────┘
                               ▼
                    ┌─────────────────────────┐
                    │ Comments to IPCS (RO)   │
                    └───────────┬─────────────┘
                                ▼
                   ┌──────────────────────────────┐
                   │ Review of comments,          │
                   │ reference cross-check;       │
                   │ preparation of Task Group    │
                   │ (TG) draft                   │
                   └───────────┬──────────────────┘
                               ▼
┌──────────┐                                      ┌──────────────┐
│ Editor   │─ ─ ─ ─ ─ ─▶ Task Group meeting ◄─ ─ ─│ Working group│
└──────────┘                   │                  │ if required  │
                               ▼                  └──────────────┘
                    ┌─────────────────────────┐
                    │ Insertion of TG changes │
                    └───────────┬─────────────┘
                                ▼
                   ┌──────────────────────────────┐
                   │ Post-TG draft; detailed      │
                   │ reference cross-check        │
                   └───────────┬──────────────────┘
                               ▼
                       ┌───────────────┐          ┌─────────────────┐
                       │   Editing     │─────────▶│ French/Spanish  │
                       └───────┬───────┘          │ translations of │
                               ▼                  │ Summary         │
┌──────────┐           ┌───────────────┐          └─────────────────┘
│ Graphics │──────────▶│ Word-processing│
└──────────┘           └───────┬───────┘
                               ▼
                       ┌───────────────┐          ┌─────────────────┐
                       │Camera-ready   │═════════▶│ Library for     │
                       │     copy      │          │ CIP Data        │
                       └───────┬───────┘          └─────────────────┘
                               ▼
                       ┌───────────────┐
                       │ Final editing │
                       └───────┬───────┘
                               ▼
                  ┌──────────────────────────┐
                  │ Approval by Director,IPCS│
                  └───────────┬──────────────┘
                              ▼
                  ┌──────────────────────────┐
                  │ WHO Publication Office   │
                  └───────────┬──────────────┘
                              ▼
             ┌─────────┐   ┌────────┐   ┌─────────────┐
             │ Printer │──▶│ Proofs │──▶│ Publication │
             └─────────┘   └────────┘   └─────────────┘

    ═══▶  routine procedure
    - -▶  optional procedure
```

The three cooperating organizations of the IPCS recognize the important role played by nongovernmental organizations. Representatives from relevant national and international associations may be invited to join the Task Group as observers. While observers may provide a valuable contribution to the process, they can only speak at the invitation of the Chairperson. Observers do not participate in the final evaluation of the chemical; this is the sole responsibility of the Task Group members. When the Task Group considers it to be appropriate, it may meet *in camera*.

All individuals who as authors, consultants or advisers participate in the preparation of the EHC monograph must, in addition to serving in their personal capacity as scientists, inform the RO if at any time a conflict of interest, whether actual or potential, could be perceived in their work. They are required to sign a conflict of interest statement. Such a procedure ensures the transparency and probity of the process.

When the Task Group has completed its review and the RO is satisfied as to the scientific correctness and completeness of the document, it then goes for language editing, reference checking, and preparation of camera-ready copy. After approval by the Director, IPCS, the monograph is submitted to the WHO Office of Publications for printing. At this time a copy of the final draft is sent to the Chairperson and Rapporteur of the Task Group to check for any errors.

It is accepted that the following criteria should initiate the updating of an EHC monograph: new data are available that would substantially change the evaluation; there is public concern for health or environmental effects of the agent because of greater exposure; an appreciable time period has elapsed since the last evaluation.

All Participating Institutions are informed, through the EHC progress report, of the authors and institutions proposed for the drafting of the documents. A comprehensive file of all comments received on drafts of each EHC monograph is maintained and is available on request. The Chairpersons of Task Groups are briefed before each meeting on their role and responsibility in ensuring that these rules are followed.

WHO TASK GROUP ON ENVIRONMENTAL HEALTH CRITERIA FOR CHRYSOTILE ASBESTOS

Members

Professor J.M. Dement, Duke Occupational Health Services, Duke University, Durham, NC, USA (*Vice-Chairperson*)[a]

Professor J.Q. Huang, Shanghai Medical University, Shanghai, China

Professor M.S. Huuskonen, Institute of Occupational Health, Helsinki, Finland[b]

Professor G. Kimizuka, Department of Pathobiology, School of Nursing, Chiba University, Chiba, Japan

Professor A. Langer, Environmental Sciences Laboratories, Brooklyn College of the City University of New York, Brooklyn, New York, USA (*Co-Rapporteur*)

Ms M.E. Meek, Priority Substances Section, Environmental Health Directorate, Health Protection Branch, Health Canada, Ottawa, Ontario, Canada (*Chairperson*)[c]

Ms M. Meldrum, Health and Safety Executive, Toxicology Unit, Bootle, United Kingdom (*Co-Rapporteur*)

---

[a] Professor J.M. Dement chaired the meeting sessions when discussions on Chapters 9, 10 and 11 were held. These sessions were held *in camera* without the presence of observers. He also chaired the final session when the whole document was adopted.

[b] Not present at the last session

[c] Not present at the discussions on Chapter 10.

Dr H. Muhle, Fraunhofer Institute for Toxicology and Aerosol Research, Hanover, Germany

Professor M. Neuberger, Institute of Environmental Hygiene, University of Vienna, Vienna, Austria

Professor J. Peto, Section of Epidemiology, Institute of Cancer Research, Royal Cancer Hospital, Sutton, Surrey, United Kingdom

Dr L. Stayner, Risk Analysis and Document Development Branch, Education and Information Division, National Institute for Occupational Safety and Health, Morgantown, West Virginia, USA

Dr V. Vu, Health and Environmental Review Division, US Environmental Protection Agency, Washington, D.C., USA

Observers

Mr D. Bouige, Asbestos International Association (AIA), Paris, France[a]

Dr G.W. Gibbs, Committee on Fibres, International Commission on Occupational Health, Spruce Grove, Alberta, Canada[b]

Secretariat

Dr Paolo Boffetta, Unit of Environmental Cancer Epidemiology, International Agency for Research on Cancer, Lyon, France

---

[a] Present only during first two days of the meeting (i.e. before the discussions on Chapters 9, 10 and 11 were held)

[b] Not present during the discussions on Chapters 9, 10 and 11, which were held *in camera*

Dr I. Fedotov, Occupational Safety and Health Branch, International Labour Office, Geneva, Switzerland

Mr Salem Milad, International Registry of Potentially Toxic Chemicals, United Nations Environment Programme, Geneva, Switzerland

Professor F. Valić, IPCS Scientific Adviser, Andrija Štampar School of Public Health, Zagreb University, Zagreb, Croatia (Responsible Officer and Secretary of Meeting)

Resource persons

Professor J. Corbett McDonald, Department of Occupational and Environmental Medicine, National Heart and Lung Institute, London, United Kingdom[a]

Professor W.J. Nicholson, Department of Community Medicine, Mount Sinai School of Medicine, New York, NY, USA

---

[a] Not present during the discussions on Chapters 9, 10 and 11, which were held *in camera*

xvii

IPCS TASK GROUP ON ENVIRONMENTAL HEALTH CRITERIA FOR CHRYSOTILE ASBESTOS

A Task Group on Environmental Health Criteria for Chrysotile Asbestos met at WHO Headquarters, Geneva, Switzerland, from 1 to 6 July 1996. Dr M. Mercier, Director IPCS, opened the Meeting and welcomed the participants on behalf of the heads of the three cooperating organizations of the IPCS (UNEP/ILO/WHO). The Task Group reviewed and revised the third draft of the monograph, made an evaluation of the risks for human health and the environment from exposure to chrysotile asbestos, and made recommendations for health protection and further research.

The first drafts were prepared by Dr G. Gibbs, Canada (Chapter 2), Mr B.J. Pigg, USA (Chapter 3), Professor W.J. Nicholson, USA (Chapter 4), Dr A. Morgan, UK and Professor M. Lippmann, USA (Chapter 5), Dr J.M.G. Davis, UK and Professor B.T. Mossman, USA (Chapter 6), Professor J.C. McDonald, UK, Professor P.J. Landrigan, USA and Professor W.J. Nicholson, USA (Chapter 7), Professor H. Schreier, Canada (Chapter 8).

In the light of international comments, the second draft was prepared under the coordination of Professor F. Valić, Croatia. Chapter 8 was modified by a group of experts in risk assessment (Professors J. Hughes, USA, J. Peto, UK, and J. Siemiatycki, Canada).

Professor F. Valić was responsible for the overall scientific content of the monograph and for the organization of the meeting, and Dr P.G. Jenkins, IPCS Central Unit, for the technical editing of the monograph.

The efforts of all who helped in the preparation and finalization of the monograph are gratefully acknowledged.

ABBREVIATIONS

ACM	asbestos-containing material
AOS	activated oxygen species
ATEM	analytical transmission electron microscopy
BAL	bronchoalveolar lavage
BP	benzo(*a*)pyrene
CI	confidence interval
EDXA	energy-dispersive X-ray analyser
f	fibre
FGF	fibroblast growth factor
LDH	lactate dehydrogenase
mpcf	millions of particles per cubic foot
mpcm	millions of particles per cubic metre
NHMI	*N*-nitrosoheptamethyleneimine
OR	odds ratio
p	particle
PCOM	phase contrast optical microscopy
PDGF	platelet-derived growth factor
PMR	proportional mortality ratio
RR	relative risk
SAED	selected area electron diffraction
SEM	scanning electron microscopy
SMR	standardized mortality ratio
TEM	transmission electron microscopy
TPA	12-O-tetradecanoylphorbol-13-acetate
TWA	time-weighted average
UICC	Union Internationale Contre le Cancer (reference asbestos samples)

INTRODUCTION

As early as 1986 the International Programme on Chemical Safety (IPCS) published the Environmental Health Criteria (EHC 53) on the health effects of natural mineral fibres with particular emphasis on asbestos (IPCS, 1986). During the next 7 years, efforts were focused on possible reduction of environmental asbestos exposure (IPCS, 1989; WHO/OCH, 1989), including the evaluation of a number of possible substitute fibres such as man-made mineral fibres (IPCS, 1988), and selected organic synthetic fibres (IPCS, 1993).

In 1992, four WHO Member States invited the Director-General of WHO to request the IPCS to update that part of EHC 53 concerning the health effects of chrysotile asbestos. The Director-General accepted the request and instructed the IPCS to develop an EHC specifically for chrysotile asbestos taking into consideration that (a) the International Labour Organisation had recommended the discontinuation of the use of crocidolite asbestos; (b) amosite asbestos was, for all practical purposes, no longer exploited; and (c) there was still wide-spread production and use of chrysotile asbestos in the world.

A number of reputable scientists (selected solely on the basis of their contributions to the open scientific literature) were approached with the request to develop individual scientific chapters for the first draft. Chapters 5, 6 and 7 were drafted by two or three authors independently. On the basis of these texts a coherent draft was prepared by the IPCS.

The drafts of chapters 5, 6 and 7 were sent for preliminary review to a limited number of recognized experts proposed by IPCS participating institutions. The full draft of the document was submitted to the standard IPCS worldwide evaluation procedure by circulating it for comments to more than 140 IPCS Contact Points.

Taking into account all the relevant comments, a second draft was developed by the IPCS. Chapter 7, drafted independently by three authors, was modified by a working group of experts and focuses on lung cancer and mesothelioma risks in populations exposed almost exclusively to chrysotile. The discussion in this chapter has been restricted primarily to direct observation from epidemiological studies.

The third draft was submitted for evaluation, modification and finalization to a Task Group of experts appointed by WHO. None of the primary authors was appointed to be a member of the Task Group.

1. SUMMARY

1.1 Identity, physical and chemical properties, sampling and analysis

Chrysotile is a fibrous hydrated magnesium silicate mineral that has been used in many commercial products. It is widely used in global commerce today. Its physical and chemical properties as a mineral are observed to vary among the exploited geological deposits. The minerals that accompany the fibre in ores are many, and among these may be some varieties of fibrous amphibole. Tremolite is thought to be especially important in this respect; its form and concentration range greatly.

Analysis of chrysotile in the workplace currently entails the use of light and electron microscopes. Various instruments and devices have been previously used to monitor environments for the presence and concentration of both total dust and fibres. The membrane filter technique and phase contrast optical microscopy are commonly used today for workplace assay (expressed as fibres per ml air); and the transmission electron microscopy is also employed. Environmental assays require the use of transmission electron microscopy. Tissue burden studies have been employed to improve information regarding exposures. Depending on the degree of attention to detail in these studies, inferences regarding mechanisms and etiology have been drawn.

Gravimetric and thermal precipitator and midget impinger techniques were previously used for workplace characterization, and these dust (not fibre) values are the only early exposure indices available for gauging exposure–response relationships. There have been many attempts to convert these values to fibres per volume of air, but these conversions have had very limited success. Conversion factors have been found to be industry-specific and even operation-specific; universal conversion factors carry high variances.

1.2 Sources of occupational and environmental exposure

Low concentrations of chrysotile are found throughout the crustal environment (air, water, ice caps and soil). Both natural and human activities contribute to fibre aerosolization and distribution. Anthropogenic sources include dusts from occupational activities, which cover ore recovery and processing, manufacturing, application, usage and, ultimately disposal.

Production occurs in 25 countries, and there are seven major producers. Annual world production of asbestos peaked at over 5 million tonnes in the mid-1970s but has since declined to a current level of about 3 million tonnes. Manufacturing of chrysotile products is undertaken in more than 100 countries, and Japan is the leading consumer country. The current main activities resulting in potential chrysotile exposure are: (a) mining and milling; (b) processing into products (friction materials, cement pipes and sheets, gaskets and seals, paper and textiles); (c) construction, repair and demolition; (d) transportation and disposal. The asbestos-cement industry is by far the largest user of chrysotile fibres, accounting for about 85% of all use.

Fibres are released during processing, installation and disposal of asbestos-containing products, as well as through normal wear of products in some instances. Manipulation of friable products may be an important source of chrysotile emission.

1.3 Occupational and environmental exposure levels

Based on data mainly from North America, Europe and Japan, in most production sectors workplace exposures in the early 1930s were very high. Levels dropped considerably to the late 1970s and have declined substantially to present day values. In the mining and milling industry in Quebec, the average fibre concentrations in air often exceeded 20 fibres/ml (f/ml) in the 1970s, while they are now generally well below 1 f/ml. In the production of asbestos-cement in Japan, typical mean concentrations were 2.5–9.5 f/ml in 1970s, while mean concentrations of 0.05–0.45 f/ml were reported in 1992. In asbestos textile manufacture in Japan, mean concentrations were

Summary

between 2.6 and 12.8 f/ml in the period between 1970 and 1975, and 0.1–0.2 f/ml in the period between 1984 and 1986. Trends have been similar in the production of friction materials: based on data available from the same country, mean concentrations of 10–35 f/ml were measured in the period between 1970 and 1975, while levels 0.2–5.5 f/ml were reported in the period between 1984 and 1986. In a plant in the United Kingdom in which a large mortality study was conducted, concentrations were generally above 20 f/ml in the period before 1931 and generally below 1 f/ml during 1970–1979.

Few data on concentrations of fibres associated with the installation and use of chrysotile-containing products are available, although this is easily the most likely place for workers to be exposed. In the maintenance of vehicles, peak concentrations of up to 16 f/ml were reported in the 1970s, while practically all measured levels after 1987 were less than 0.2 f/ml. Time-weighted average exposures during passenger vehicle repair in the 1980s were generally less than 0.05 f/ml. However, with no controls, blowing off debris from drums resulted in short-term high concentrations of dust.

There is potential for exposure of maintenance personnel to mixed asbestos fibre types due to large quantities of friable asbestos in place. In buildings with control plans, personal exposure of building maintenance personnel in the USA, expressed as 8-h time-weighted averages, was between 0.002 and 0.02 f/ml. These values are of the same order of magnitude as typical exposures during telecommunication switchwork (0.009 f/ml) and above-ceiling work (0.037 f/ml), although higher concentrations were reported in utility space work (0.5 f/ml). Concentrations may be considerably higher where no control plans have been introduced. In one case, short-term episodic concentrations were 1.6 f/ml during sweeping and 15.5 f/ml during dusting of library books in a building with a very friable chrysotile-containing surface formulation. Most other 8-h time-weighted averages are about two orders of magnitude less.

Based on surveys conducted before 1986, fibre concentrations (fibres > 5 μm in length) in outdoor air, measured in Austria, Canada, Germany, South Africa and the USA, ranged between 0.0001 and about 0.01 f/ml, levels in most samples being less than 0.001 f/ml.

Means or medians were between 0.00005 and 0.02 f/ml, based on more recent determinations in Canada, Italy, Japan, the Slovak Republic, Switzerland, United Kingdom and USA.

Fibre concentrations in public buildings, even those with friable asbestos-containing materials, are within the range of those measured in ambient air. Concentrations (fibres > 5 µm in length) in buildings in Germany and Canada reported before 1986 were generally less than 0.002 f/ml. In more recent surveys in Belgium, Canada, the Slovak Republic, United Kingdom and USA, mean values were between 0.00005 and 0.0045 f/ml. Only 0.67% of chrysotile fibres were longer than 5 µm.

1.4 Uptake, clearance, retention and translocation

The deposition of inhaled chrysotile asbestos is dependent upon the aerodynamic diameter, the length and the morphology of the fibre. Most airborne chrysotile fibres are considered respirable because their fibre diameters are less than 3 µm, equal to an aerodynamic diameter of about 10 µm. In laboratory rats, chrysotile fibres are deposited primarily at alveolar duct bifurcations.

In the nasopharyngeal and tracheobronchial regions, chrysotile fibres are cleared via mucocilliary clearance. At the alveolar duct bifurcations the fibres are taken up by epithelial cells. Fibre length is an important determinant of alveolar clearance of chrysotile fibres. There is extensive evidence from animal studies that short fibres (less than 5 µm long) are cleared more rapidly than long fibres (longer than 5 µm). The mechanisms of the relatively more rapid clearance of chrysotile fibres compared to those of amphiboles are not completely known. It has been hypothesized that short chrysotile fibres are cleared through phagocytosis by alveolar macrophages, while long chrysotile fibres are cleared mainly by breakage and/or dissolution. To what extent chrysotile fibres are translocated to the interstitium, pleural tissue and other extrathoracic tissues is not fully understood.

Analyses of human lungs of workers exposed to chrysotile asbestos indicate much greater retention of tremolite, an amphibole asbestos commonly associated with commercial chrysotile in small

Summary

proportions, than of chrysotile. The more rapid removal of chrysotile fibres from the human lung is further supported by findings from animal studies showing that chrysotile is more rapidly cleared from the lung than are amphiboles including crocidolite and amosite.

Available data from studies in humans and animals are insufficient to evaluate the possible uptake, distribution and excretion of chrysotile fibres from ingestion. Available evidence indicates that, if penetration of chrysotile fibres across the gut wall does occur, it is extremely limited. One study indicated an increased level of chrysotile fibres in the urine of workers occupationally exposed to chrysotile.

1.5 Effects on animals and cells

Various experimental samples of chrysotile fibres have been shown in numerous long-term inhalation studies to cause fibrogenic and carcinogenic effects in laboratory rats. These effects include interstitial fibrosis and cancer of the lung and pleura. In most cases, there appears to be an association between fibrosis and tumours in the rat lung. Fibrogenic and carcinogenic effects have also been found in long-term animal studies (mainly in rats) using other modes of administration (e.g., intratracheal instillation and intrapleural or intraperitoneal injection).

Exposure/dose–response relationships for chrysotile-induced pulmonary fibrosis, lung cancer and mesothelioma have not been adequately investigated in long-term animal inhalation studies. Inhalation studies conducted to date, mainly using a single exposure concentration, show fibrogenic and carcinogenic responses at airborne fibre concentrations ranging from 100 to a few thousand fibres/ml. When data from various studies are combined, there appears to be a relationship between airborne fibre concentrations and lung cancer incidence. This type of analysis, however, may not be scientifically sound as different experimental conditions were used in available studies.

In non-inhalation experiments (intrapleural and intraperitoneal injection studies), dose–response relationships for mesothelioma have been demonstrated for chrysotile fibres. Data from these types of studies, however, may not be suitable for the evaluations of human risk from inhalation exposure to fibres.

Tremolite asbestos, a minor component mineral of commercial chrysotile, has also been shown to be carcinogenic and fibrogenic in a single inhalation experiment and an intraperitoneal injection study in rats. Exposure/dose–response data are not available to allow direct comparison of the cancer potency of tremolite and chrysotile.

The ability of fibres to induce fibrogenic and carcinogenic effects appears to be dependent on their individual characteristics, including fibre dimension and durability (i.e. biopersistence in target tissues), which are determined in part by the physico-chemical properties. It has been well documented in experimental studies that short fibres (shorter than 5 µm) are less biologically active than long fibres (longer than 5 µm). It is still uncertain, however, whether short fibres have any significant biological activity. Furthermore, it is not known how long a fibre needs to remain in the lung in order to induce preneoplastic effects, since the appearance of asbestos-related cancer generally occurs later in the animal's life.

The mechanisms by which chrysotile and other fibres cause fibrogenic and carcinogenic effects are not completely understood. Possible mechanisms of fibrogenic effects of fibres include chronic inflammation process mediated by production of growth factors (e.g., TNF-alpha) and reactive oxygen species. With regard to fibre-induced carcinogenicity, several hypotheses have been proposed. These include: DNA damage by reactive oxygen species induced by fibres; direct DNA damage by physical interactions between fibres and target cells; enhancement of cell proliferation by fibres; fibre-provoked chronic inflammatory reactions leading to prolonged release of lysozymal enzymes, reactive oxygen species, cytokines and growth factors; and action by fibres as co-carcinogens or carriers of chemical carcinogens to the target tissues. It is likely, however, that all these mechanisms contribute to the carcinogenicity of chrysotile fibres, as such effects have been observed in various *in vitro* systems of human and mammalian cells.

Summary

Overall, the available toxicological data provide clear evidence that chrysotile fibres can cause fibrogenic and carcinogenic hazard to humans. The data, however, are not adequate for providing quantitative estimates of the risk to humans. This is because there are inadequate exposure–response data from inhalation studies, and there are uncertainties concerning the sensitivities of the animal studies for predicting human risk.

Chrysotile fibres have been tested in several oral carcinogenicity studies. Carcinogenic effects have not been reported in available studies.

1.6 Effects on humans

Commercial grades of chrysotile have been associated with an increased risk of pneumoconiosis, lung cancer and mesothelioma in numerous epidemiological studies of exposed workers.

The non-malignant diseases associated with exposure to chrysotile comprise a somewhat complex mixture of clinical and pathological syndromes not readily definable for epidemiological study. The prime concern has been asbestosis, generally implying a disease associated with diffuse interstitial pulmonary fibrosis accompanied by varying degrees of pleural involvement.

Studies of workers exposed to chrysotile in different sectors have broadly demonstrated exposure–response or exposure–effect relationships for chrysotile-induced asbestosis, in so far as increasing levels of exposure have produced increases in the incidence and severity of disease. However, there are difficulties in defining this relationship, due to factors such as uncertainties in diagnosis and the possibility of disease progression on cessation of exposure.

Furthermore, some variation in risk estimates are evident among the available studies. The reasons for the variations are not entirely clear, but may relate to uncertainties in exposure estimates, airborne fibre size distributions in the various industry sectors and statistical models. Asbestotic changes are common following prolonged exposures of 5 to 20 f/ml.

The overall relative risks for lung cancer are generally not elevated in the studies of workers in asbestos-cement production and in some of the cohorts of asbestos-cement production workers. The exposure–response relationship between chrysotile and lung cancer risk appears to be 10–30 times higher in studies of textile workers than in studies of workers in mining and milling industries. The relative risks of lung cancer in the textile manufacturing sector in relation to estimated cumulative exposure are, therefore, some 10–30 times greater than those observed in chrysotile mining. The reasons for this variation in risk are not clear, so several hypotheses, including variations in fibre size distribution, have been proposed.

Estimation of the risk of mesothelioma is complicated in epidemiological studies by factors such as the rarity of the disease, the lack of mortality rates in the populations used as reference, and problems in diagnosis and reporting. In many cases, therefore, risks have not been calculated, and cruder indicators have been used, such as absolute numbers of cases and deaths, and ratios of mesothelioma over lung cancers or total deaths.

Based on data reviewed in this monograph, the largest number of mesotheliomas has occurred in the chrysotile mining and milling sector. All the observed 38 cases were pleural with the exception of one of low diagnostic probability, which was pleuro-peritoneal. None occurred in workers exposed for less than 2 years. There was a clear dose–response relationship, with crude rates of mesotheliomas (cases/ 1000 person-years) ranging from 0.15 for those with cumulative exposure less than 3530 million particles per m^3 (mpcm)-years (< 100 million particles per cubic foot (mpcf)-years) to 0.97 for those with exposures of more than 10 590 mpcm-years (> 300 mpcf-years).

Proportions of deaths attributable to mesotheliomas in cohort studies in the various mining and production sectors range from 0 to 0.8%. Caution should be exercised in interpreting these proportions as studies do not provide comparable data stratifying deaths by exposure intensity, duration of exposure or time since first exposure.

There is evidence that fibrous tremolite causes mesothelioma in humans. Since commercial chrysotile may contain fibrous tremolite, it has been hypothesized that the latter may contribute to the induction of mesotheliomas in some populations exposed primarily to chrysotile. The extent to which the observed excesses of mesothelioma might be attributed to the fibrous tremolite content has not been resolved.

The epidemiological evidence that chrysotile exposure is associated with an increased risk for cancer sites other than the lung or pleura is inconclusive. There is limited information on this issue for chrysotile *per se*, although there is some inconsistent evidence for an association between asbestos exposure (all forms) and laryngeal, kidney and gastrointestinal tract cancers. A significant excess of stomach cancer has been observed in a study of Quebec chrysotile miners and millers, but possible confounding by diet, infections or other risk factors has not been addressed.

It should be recognized that although the epidemiological studies of chrysotile-exposed workers have been primarily limited to the mining and milling, and manufacturing sector, there is evidence, based on the historical pattern of disease associated with exposure to mixed fibre types in western countries, that risks are likely to be greater among workers in construction and possibly other user industries.

1.7 Environmental fate and effects on biota

Serpentine outcroppings occur world-wide. Mineral components, including chrysotile, are eroded through crustal processes and are transported to become a component of the water cycle, sediment population and soil profile. Chrysotile presence and concentrations have been measured in water, air and other units of the crust.

Chrysotile and its associated serpentine minerals chemically degrade at the surface. This produces profound changes in soil pH and introduces a variety of trace metals into the environment. This has in turn produced measurable effects on plant growth, soil biota (including microbes and insects), fish and invertebrates. Some data indicate that grazing animals (sheep and cattle) undergo changes in blood chemistry following ingestion of grasses grown on serpentine outcrops.

2. IDENTITY, PHYSICAL AND CHEMICAL PROPERTIES, SAMPLING AND ANALYSIS

2.1 Identity

2.1.1 Chemical composition

Chrysotile, referred to as white asbestos, is a naturally occurring fibrous hydrated magnesium silicate belonging to the serpentine group of minerals. The chemical composition, crystal structure and polytypic forms of the serpentine minerals have been described by Langer & Nolan (1994).

The composition of chrysotile is close to the ideal unit cell formula ($Mg_3Si_2O_5(OH)_4$); substitution by other elements in the crystal structure is possible. According to Skinner et al. (1988) substitution possibilities are:

$$(Mg_{3-x-y} R_x^{+2} R_y^{+3})(Si_{2-y} R_y^{+3})O_5 (OH)_4,$$

where $R^{2+} = Fe^{2+}$, Mn^{2+} or Ni^{2+} and $R^{3+}=Al^{3+}$ or Fe^{3+}.

Results of a typical chemical analysis are shown in Table 1 of Environmental Health Criteria 53 (IPCS, 1986).

Trace amounts of some other elements, such as Na, Ca and K, are probably due to the presence of other minerals admixed in the ore (see section 2.1.6).

2.1.2 Structure

Chrysotile is a sheet silicate with a basic building block of $(Si_2O_5)_n$ in which three of the oxygen atoms in each tetrahedron base are shared with adjacent tetrahedra in the same layer. The apical oxygens of the tetrahedra in the silica sheet become a component member of the overlying brucite layer ($Mg(OH)_2$) (Speil & Leineweber, 1969). As the dimensions of the cations in the silica and brucite sheets are different, strain is produced, which is accommodated by the formation of a scroll structure. Yada (1967) produced transmission electron micrographs that permitted visualization of this morphological feature. The curvature occurs with the brucite layer on the outer surface. The resulting capillaries are common to most specimens although solid cores have been found.

When more than one structure occurs, they are called polytypes: orthochrysotile (orthorhombic structure), clinochrysotile (monoclinic structure) and parachrysotile (cylindrical or polygonal Povlen-type structures) (Wicks, 1979). Most chrysotile is a mixture of the ortho- and clino-polytypes in various proportions (Speil & Leineweber, 1969).

2.1.3 Fibre forms in the ore

Chrysotile can occur in the host rock as "cross-fibre" (fibre axes at right angles to the seam or vein), "slip-fibre" (fibre axes parallel to the seam) or massive fibre (in which there is no recognizable fibre orientation, as in the New Idria deposit in USA).

2.1.4 Fibre properties

Depending on the relative flexibility, fibres may be "harsh" or "soft". Chrysotile fibres generally occur with properties between these end-types (Badollet, 1948). While amphibole fibres are generally harsh, most chrysotile fibres are soft, although fibres displaying intermediate properties also occur. Harshness has been reported to be related to the water content of the fibre, i.e. the higher the water content the "softer" the fibre (Woodroofe, 1956), relative contents of clino- and ortho-chrysotile, and the presence of fine mineral intergrowth (Speil & Leineweber, 1969).

Harsh chrysotile fibres tend to be straighter and less flexible than the soft fibres. Inhalation of respirable straight fibres is reported to be associated with greater penetration to the terminal bronchioles than in the case of "curly" fibres (Timbrell, 1965, 1970).

The fibres can be classified into crude chrysotile (hand-selected fibres in essentially native or unfiberized form) and milled fibres (after mechanical treatment of the ore). Fibre grades used for different products vary from country to country. The Canadian system has been described by Cossette & Delvaux (1979). The Canadian grading system is widely used internationally.

At the turn of this century, the fibres of major commercial importance were several centimetres long. With time, as new applications developed, shorter fibres became important. This change is likely to have altered the nature of exposure in some circumstances.

2.1.5 UICC samples

Two UICC (Union Internationale Contre le Cancer) standard reference samples of chrysotile asbestos were available for use in experimental work. One was from Zimbabwe (Chrysotile A) and the other was a composite sample of fibres from Canadian mines in the eastern townships of Quebec (Chrysotile B). The physico-chemical properties of these samples are well characterized and details of their composition and properties have been reported (Timbrell et al., 1968; Rendall, 1970). These mixtures were artificial and did not reflect any one commercially available fibre.

2.1.6 Associated minerals in chrysotile ore

The mineral dusts to which miners or millers might be exposed are determined by the minerals associated with each of the chrysotile ore deposits. These depend on the composition of the original rock types and on the materials added or removed during geological events, surface weathering processes, etc. The spacial relationships among these components within ore bodies vary significantly from deposit to deposit.

Iron is ubiquitous in chrysotile deposits derived from ultramafic rocks. In some of these, magnetite occurs in intimate association with the fibres (e.g., in Quebec). In other deposits types, e.g., in carbonate rocks, the iron content is low (e.g., in Arizona). Brucite, or nemalite (the fibrous form of brucite), is found in some deposits. Micas, feldspars, altered feldspars, talc and carbonate minerals may be present. Langer & Nolan (1994) listed minerals likely to be associated with ultramafic rocks in which chrysotile is found, and Gibbs (1971a) listed more than 70 minerals occurring in the Quebec chrysotile mining region. Minerals such as magnetite, calcite and zeolites may also occur in a fibrous form.

Amphiboles may also be encountered, some in fibrous form. These latter minerals have been found in studies of lung tissues of exposed workers. Tremolite, ferro-tremolite, actinolite, anthophyllite and other amphibole minerals have been described. Their occurrence in ore bodies is both heterogeneous in distribution and variable in concentration. Addison & Davies (1990) found tremolite in 28 out of 81 ore samples (34.6%) at concentrations (when detected) from 0.01 to about 0.6%. The average concentration was about 0.09%. The form of the amphibole, whether asbestos or massive, was not given. This information may be crucial in considering the mineral type as an agent of disease, especially for mesothelioma.

Trace metals have been described in association with fibres, particularly chromium, cobalt, nickel, iron and manganese (Cralley et al., 1967; Gibbs, 1971a; Morgan & Cralley, 1973; Oberdörster et al., 1980). Concentrations in mills in the late 1960s were several times higher than those measured at textile plants at that time (Gibbs, 1971a).

Naturally occurring chrysotile has been shown to contain trace quantities of organic compounds, predominantly straight-chain alkanes (Gibbs, 1971b). Processed fibres may also contain organic compounds including polycyclic aromatic hydrocarbons (Gibbs, 1971a; Gibbs & Hui, 1971). Concentrations of polycyclic aromatic hydrocarbons in the air of chrysotile mills were found to be lower than levels in urban areas (Gibbs, 1971a). Fibres can also be contaminated by alkanes and by antioxidants from storage in polyethylene bags (Commins & Gibbs, 1969; Gibbs & Hui, 1971).

Radon concentrations in the Quebec chrysotile mines were reported to be below 0.3 Standard Working Level (Gibbs, 1971a). This has been rejected as an agent of disease among miners, especially for lung cancer.

2.2 Physical and chemical properties

The mineralogy and properties of chrysotile have been summarized by Wicks (1979), Pooley (1987), and Langer & Nolan (1994).

2.2.1 Physical properties

The physical properties of chrysotile, as they affect human health, have been described in Langer & Nolan (1986, 1994) and IPCS (1986).

Harshness has been discussed in section 2.1.4.

Heating of chrysotile fibre at 700 °C for an hour converts it to an amorphous, anhydrous magnesium silicate material (Speil & Leineweber, 1969). Intensive dry grinding also destroys the structure of chrysotile. Analysis of wear debris from brake linings made with asbestos has shown that virtually all of the chrysotile fibre is converted to amorphous material, in association with the mineral forsterite (a recrystallization product). The conversion is explained by localized temperatures above 1000 °C at the point of contact between the brake lining and the drum (Lynch, 1968; Rowson, 1978; Williams & Muhlbaier, 1982). The fibres found in the brake wear debris are predominantly (99%) less than 0.4 µm in length (Rohl et al., 1977; Williams & Muhlbaier, 1982). Rodelsperger et al. (1986) found less than 1% of fibres longer than 5 µm.

Size and shape are the most important characteristics for defining the respirability of fibres. For workplace regulatory purposes a fibre has been defined most frequently as having an aspect ratio (ratio of fibre length to fibre diameter) of at least 3:1. Regulatory definitions usually impose a length of 5 µm or greater for workplace assay.

Chrysotile bundles may be split longitudinally to form thinner fibres. The ultimate fibre is called a fibril. Yada (1967), by means of high resolution transmission electron microscopy, showed that basic spiral elements of chrysotile consist of 5 silica-magnesia units with approximately 10 silica-magnesia units forming the 0.007 µm wall of a single fibril. The diameter of the ultimate fibril is about 0.03 µm.

The fibres of significance in health risk evaluation are those that can be inhaled. Timbrell (1970, 1973) showed that chrysotile fibres less than about 3.5 µm in diameter can enter the conducting airways of the lung. The radius of curvature of the chrysotile fibre may play a role in the ability of a fibre to penetrate to distant sites along the conducting airways.

As it is possible to have long narrow fibres and short narrow fibres, descriptions of fibrous aerosols by "mean or median diameter", or "mean or median length" do not provide sufficient information. Comparisons of fibrous aerosols to which subjects are exposed may therefore be limited. The measurements of dimensions are time-consuming and complete data sets are scant.

Results of most distributions reported are incomplete. Unless specific steps have been taken to evaluate very long fibres, transmission electron microscopy (TEM) will understate the number of long fibres (>20 µm). Because the proportion of very long fibres is low, random scanning rarely encounters them. Scanning electron microscopy (SEM) usually requires coating of the specimen. Most preparation techniques obscure single chrysotile fibrils. In addition, if chemical analysis of individual fibres is not made, other fibres may be erroneously reported as chrysotile.

It has been noted that the vast majority of airborne chrysotile fibres are short, the percentage of fibres more than 5 µm long in mining and milling being about 1.3 and 4.1%, respectively (Gibbs & Hwang, 1980), while data show that up to 24% of fibres may be longer than 5 µm in certain textile spinning operations (Gibbs, 1994). Virtually all airborne fibres have a diameter of less than 3 µm and are thus respirable.

The cross-section of a chrysotile fibril is approximately circular (see figure in Yada, 1967). This is important in calculating the mass of individual fibres. Generally, the surface area depends on the degree of fibre openness. The New Idria (Coalinga) material has a surface area of about 78 m^2/g and an average fibril diameter of 0.0275 µm, while the Canadian 7R has a surface area of about 50 m^2/g and an average fibril diameter of 0.0375 µm (Speil & Leineweber, 1969). It has been suggested that surface area plays a role in imparting biological potential.

Timbrell (1975) reported the magnetic properties of fibres. Chrysotile showed no preferred orientation in magnetic fields.

It has been observed that industrial processing of fibres from different sources may affect total airborne dust concentrations.

2.2.2 Chemical properties

Chrysotile exhibits significant solubility in aqueous neutral or acidic environments (Langer & Pooley, 1973; Jaurand et al., 1977; Spurny, 1982). In contact with dilute acids or aqueous medium at pH less than 10, magnesium leaches from the outer brucite layer (Nagy & Bates, 1952; Atkinson, 1973; Morgan & Cralley, 1973). Magnesium loss has also been demonstrated *in vivo*. The surface area of leached chrysotile is greatly increased (Badollet & Gannt, 1965). The solubility of the outer brucite layer of chrysotile in body fluids greatly affects bioaccumulation in lung tissues. The role of chemical properties in the biological behaviour of chrysotile has been recently discussed (Langer & Nolan, 1986, 1994).

The adsorption of polar organic agents on the surface of chrysotile is reported to be higher than that of less polar or non-polar agents (Speil & Leineweber, 1969; Gorski & Stettler, 1974). The binding of carcinogens such as benzo(*a*)pyrene, nitrosonornicotine and *N*-acetyl-2-aminofluorene to chrysotile has been studied by Harvey et al. (1984). Adsorption of components of cigarette smoke onto the surface of chrysotile fibres has been suggested to play a role in the etiology of lung cancer in fibre-exposed cigarette smokers. The fibre may act as a vehicle which transports polycyclic aromatic hydrocarbons across membranes of the target cells (Gerde & Scholander, 1989).

2.3 Sampling and analytical methods

The collection of samples from air, water, biological specimens, soils or sediments must follow an appropriate sampling strategy. A

Identity, Physical and Chemical Properties

review of methods for sampling asbestos fibres has been published (IPCS, 1986).

The most commonly used analytical methods involve phase-contrast optical microscopy (PCOM) (in the workplace) and transmission electron microscopy (TEM) (in the general environment). PCOM is resolution-limited and non-specific for fibre characterization. TEM overcomes both limitations (Dement & Wallingford, 1990).

2.3.1 Workplace sampling

The most widely used method for the last 20 years has been the membrane filter method. Several attempts have been made to standardize the method (CEC, 1983; ILO, 1984; AIA, 1988; NIOSH, 1989a; ISO, 1993). A recommended method for the determination of airborne fibre concentration by PCOM (membrane filter method) has been published (WHO, 1997).

A known volume of air is drawn through a membrane filter on which the number of fibres is determined using a phase contrast microscope (see section 2.3.3.2). Special attention should be given to flow rates, sampling time, face velocity through the filter, and where, when and how to sample. Preference should be given to assessing individual exposure by personal sampling. The sampling strategy should be selected to yield the best estimate of an 8-h time-weighted average concentration. Excursions may be evaluated for regulatory purposes. If the purpose of the measurement is evaluation of control measures, other methods may also be used.

2.3.2 Sampling in the general environment

Methods for sampling ambient air depend on the method of analysis, but generally involve filtering airborne particles from relatively large volumes of air using membrane filters. Strategies and sampling methods have been described by Rood (1991) and reviewed in detail in the Health Effects Institute study of asbestos in public buildings (HEI, 1991).

EHC 203: Chrysotile asbestos

For analysis of water, sample specimens are collected and filtered through polycarbonate filters. If there is much organic debris, this must be removed to improve particle detection. The fibres must be re-prepared before analysis. The instrumental method is the same as that used for air samples.

2.3.3 Analytical methods

Analyses are performed to identify the fibre or fibres present and to determine their concentrations.

2.3.3.1 Fibre identification

Several methods have been developed to identify chrysotile asbestos using dispersion staining methods and polarization microscopy (Julian & McCrone, 1970; McCrone, 1978; Churchyard & Copeland, 1988; NIOSH, 1989a). NIOSH (1989b) described the procedure specifically for the analysis of asbestos bulk samples.

The limit of visibility of fibres, depending on the microscope and light source used, is in the range 0.2-0.3 µm. With most high quality research microscopes, chrysotile fibres of 0.22 µm are generally reported as being observable. The experience and expertise of the microscopist and the quality of the laboratory set-up both influence the outcome.

Fibres with diameters less than about 0.22 µm cannot be seen with a light optical microscope. When fibres with diameters less than this value need to be analysed, TEM is used. This method is generally applied to the identification and characterization of fibres in water and in ambient air (Chatfield, 1979, 1987; Rood, 1991; ISO, 1991; HEI, 1991). The most reliable method of identifying chrysotile fibres is the combination of morphology, chemistry and electron diffraction (Skikne et al., 1971; Langer & Pooley, 1973). Several methods for the determination of amphibole fibres in chrysotile have been described (Addison & Davies, 1990).

Analytical methods using scanning electron microscopy (SEM) have also been developed (AIA, 1984; WHO, 1985; ISO, 1992).

Identity, Physical and Chemical Properties

2.3.3.2 *Measurement of airborne fibre concentrations*

a) Workplace

In the PCOM method, the membrane filter is dissolved or collapsed using a solvent with a refractive index which matches the refractive index of the filter medium, rendering it invisible. Fibres entrained on the filter are made readily visible.

The number of fibres of specified length and diameter in a known area of the filter is counted at magnifications of 400 to 500. A graticule has been designed for this purpose. Development of the HSE/NPL slide (LeGuen et al., 1984), which permits laboratories to standardize the limit of visibility of their microscopes and microscopists, has improved the potential for interlaboratory agreement in counts.

Improvements in the mounting techniques and counting strategy has resulted in higher fibre counts than those found using the same techniques in the early 1970s (HSE, 1979; Gibbs, 1994). This change was estimated in the United Kingdom to cause a two-fold increase in the reported fibre concentrations (HSE, 1979).

Instrumentation for automatic counting has been developed (e.g., Kenny, 1984) but has failed to receive wide international recognition.

b) Ambient air

The diameter of most chrysotile fibres found in the non-occupational environment is below the resolution of the light optical microscope (Rooker et al., 1982).

The most reliable method for determining the concentration of chrysotile fibres in ambient air is TEM. Most currently available transmission electron microscopes have a resolution of about 0.2 nm; in combination with an energy-dispersive X-ray analyser (EDXA), TEM can chemically characterize fibres down to a diameter of 0.01 µm. The disadvantage of TEM is the small area that can be scanned when employing very high magnifications. This makes analysis of the long fibres (>5 µm) more limited in accuracy (Coin et al., 1992). A review of the use of TEM and a comparison of direct and indirect methods of filter preparation have been published recently (HEI, 1991).

SEM has been used in the measurement of chrysotile. Most SEMs have a resolution intermediate between that of TEM and PCOM.

2.3.3.3 Lung tissue analysis

Several methods have been described (Langer & Pooley, 1973; Gaudichet et al., 1980; Rogers et al., 1991a,b). All methods use ashing or digestion of tissues, TEM, SAED and EDXA. International standardization of these methods has not as yet been carried out. For this reason comparison of results from different laboratories is often difficult to make.

2.3.3.4 Gravimetric analysis

Gravimetric methods have been applied in some countries for the evaluation of workplace conditions and emissions (Rickards, 1973; Middleton, 1982). Relatively large samples of dust are needed and the methods do not distinguish between the fibres and non-fibrous dusts nor among mineral components of each group. In view of this and the current belief that counts of fibres better define the health risk, gravimetric methods are limited in application. However, it must also be recognized that bulk dust assay is a useful index for control evaluation and should be used if membrane filter techniques are unavailable.

2.4 Conversion factors

The concentrations of airborne chrysotile fibres in the workplace are expressed as the number of fibres per millilitre (f/ml) of air, fibres per litre (f/litre) of air or fibres per cubic metre (f/m^3) of air, or in milligrams per cubic metre (mg/m^3) of air. Concentrations are expressed as number of fibres per cubic metre or nanograms per cubic metre (ng/m^3) in the general environment.

Identity, Physical and Chemical Properties

The number of fibres per millilitre, obtained by the method of membrane filtration and PCOM, is currently used by regulatory agencies in most countries for the workplace. It is for this reason that the conversion of results obtained by different methods into membrane filter equivalents has been performed. Critiques of such conversions have been published (Walton, 1982; Valić, 1993; Gibbs, 1994).

2.4.1 Conversion from airborne particle to fibre concentrations

In almost all epidemiological studies in which health effects have been related to exposure, concentration measurements were made using methods quite different from the membrane filter technique. The early instruments employed were the thermal precipitator in the United Kingdom, and the midget impinger in North America. Gravimetric measurements have also been used.

Attempts to convert the midget impinger count to an equivalent membrane filter fibre count have shown that no single conversion factor applies. Large variations in the ratios of midget impinger to membrane filter counts occur in different industries, between jobs within a single industry, or at a single plant site (Ayer et al., 1965; Gibbs & Lachance, 1974). Similar conversion problems were encountered in other countries where attempts were made to convert konimeter or thermal precipitator results to membrane filter equivalents (DuToit & Gilfillan, 1979; DuToit et al., 1983; Valić & Cigula, 1992).

Side-by-side study of conversion factors has shown the correlation between particle and fibre counts to be limited. Both industry and operation-specific correlations have been made but are only site-specific. Although some comparisons made for epidemiological studies have yielded valuable data, no universal factor has ever been found. High variance exists. Temporal change in dust conditions in plants may have also affected conversion factors (Dagbert, 1976). The range of conversion ratios between work sites has been large (Doll & Peto, 1985). For purposes of exposure–response studies, conversions based on industry- and operation-specific data have proven valuable in some instances.

2.4.2 Conversion from total mass to fibre number concentrations

The conversions from total mass concentrations of dust determined gravimetrically into the fibre number concentrations may also be generally subject to great errors (Pott, 1978; IPCS, 1986). However, in some specific industries a good correlation has been achieved (Fei & Huang, 1989; Huang, 1990).

When measurements of airborne fibre concentrations are made using transmission electron microscopy, determination of fibre lengths and diameters are necessary. If chrysotile is split into fibrils, approximate mass can be calculated by determining the fibre dimensions and using fibre density in the calculation.

3. SOURCES OF OCCUPATIONAL AND ENVIRONMENTAL EXPOSURE

3.1 Natural occurrence

Chrysotile is present in most serpentine rock formations. As a result, chrysotile originating from serpentine rock is often found in air and water due to natural weathering (Nicholson & Pundsack, 1973; Neuberger et al., 1996).

Workable deposits are present in over 40 countries. Twenty-five of these currently produce chrysotile. Canada, South Africa, Russia and Zimbabwe have 90% of the established world reserves (Shride, 1973).

Chrysotile is emitted from both natural and industrial sources. No measurements concerning the extent of release of airborne fibres through natural weathering processes are available. A study of the mineral content of the Greenland ice cap showed that airborne chrysotile existed long before it was used commercially on a large scale. Ice core dating showed the presence of chrysotile as early as 1750 (Bowes et al., 1977).

Chrysotile is introduced into water by the weathering of chrysotile-containing rocks and ores, in addition to the effects of industrial effluents and atmospheric pollution (Canada Environmental Health Directorate, 1979). The largest concentrations of asbestos in drinking-water generally occur from erosion of asbestos deposits (Polissar, 1993; Neuberger et al., 1996). Millette JR ed. (1983) has attributed chrysotile in water supplies to erosion from natural sources in areas such as San Francisco, Sherbrooke and Seattle. Millette et al. (1980) have shown that in the USA asbestos in drinking-water is primarily chrysotile.

3.2 Anthropogenic sources

Chrysotile was at one time used in many applications, which included both friable and non-friable products (Shride, 1973). Currently, the human activities resulting in potential chrysotile exposure can be divided into broad categories: (a) mining and milling, (b) processing of asbestos into products (such as friction materials, cement pipe and sheet, gaskets and seals, paper and textiles), (c) construction and repair activities, and (d) transportation and, especially, disposal of chrysotile-containing waste products.

Chrysotile is by far the predominant asbestos fibre consumed today, e.g., in the USA 98.5% asbestos consumption in 1992 was chrysotile (Pigg, 1994).

3.2.1 Production

Although there are 25 countries currently producing chrysotile, seven countries account for the major part of world production (Brazil, Canada, China, Kazakhstan, Russia, South Africa and Zimbabwe) (US Department of Interior, 1993).

World production of asbestos increased 50% between 1964 and 1973 when it reached 5 million tonnes (US Department of Interior, 1991), but production has generally declined since the mid-1970s to its current level of 3.1 million tonnes. Table 1 shows the yearly production levels by countries between 1988 and 1992.

Table 2 shows the decline in major asbestos uses in the USA during the period 1977–1991 (US Department of Interior, 1986, 1991).

Chrysotile ore is usually mined in open-pit operations. Possible sources of emissions are drilling, blasting, loading broken rock and transporting ore to the primary crusher or waste sites. Subsequently, the ore is crushed and emissions may result during unloading, primary crushing, screening, secondary crushing, conveying and stockpiling. A drying step follows, involving conveying the ore to the dryer building, screening, drying, tertiary crushing, conveying ore to dry rock storage building and dry rock storage. The next step is the milling of the ore. In well-controlled mills, this is largely confined in the mill building, and presents low emissions because the mill air is collected and ducted through control devices (US EPA, 1986). In poorly controlled mills the emissions may be high.

Table 1. World production, of asbestos (tonnes)[a] (from: US Department of Interior, 1993)

Country[b]	1988	1989	1990	1991	1992
Argentina	2328	225	300[e]	250[e]	50
Bosnia & Herzegovina[c]	–	–	–	–	1000
Brazil	227 653	206 195	232 332[f]	233 100[f]	233 000
Bulgaria	300	300	500[f]	500[e,f]	500
Canada	710 357	701 227	685 627	689 000[f]	585 000
China[e]	150 000[f]	181 000[f]	221 000[f]	230 000	240 000
Columbia[e, d]	7600	7900	8000	8000	8000
Cyprus	14 585	–	–	–	–
Egypt	166	312	369	450[f]	450
Greece	71 114	73 300[f]	65 993[f]	5500[e,f]	–
India	31 123	36 502	26 053[f]	24 094[f]	25 000
Iran[e]	3410[f,g]	3300	2800[f]	3000[f]	3000
Italy	94 549	44 348	3862	3000[e,f]	1500
Japan[e]	5000	5000	5000	5000	5000
Kazakhstan[f]	–	–	–	–	300 000
Korea	2428	2361	1534	1500[e]	1600
Russia	–	–	–	–	1 400 000

25

Table 1 (contd).

Country[b]	1988	1989	1990	1991	1992
Serbia & Montenegro[c]	–	–	–	–	1700
South Africa	145 678	156 594	145 791	148 525[r]	123 951[g]
Swaziland	22 804	27 291	35 938	13 888[r]	35 000
Turkey	50[e]	–	–	–	–
Former-USSR[e]	2 600 000	2 600 000	2 400 000	2 000 000	–
USA (sold or used by producers)	18 233	17 427	W	20 061	15 573
Former-Yugoslavia	17 030	9111	6578	5500[e]	–
Zimbabwe	186 581	187 006[r]	160 861[r]	141 697[r]	140 000
Total	4 310 989[r]	4 259 399	4 002 538[r]	3 533 065[r]	3 120 524

[a] Marketable fibre production. Table includes data available until 19 April 1993
[b] In addition to the countries listed, Afghanistan, Czechoslovakia, North Korea and Romania also produce asbestos, but output is not officially reported, and available general information is inadequate for the formulation of reliable estimates of output levels.
[c] Formerly part of Yugoslavia; data were not reported separately until 1992.
[d] Estimated fibre production (in tonnes), based on reported crude production, was as follows: 1988: 152 896; 1989:-158 149; 1990: 159 600; 1991: 160 332; 1992: 160 000 (estimated).
[e] Estimated
[f] Formerly part of the USSR; data were not reported separately until 1992.
[g] Reported figure.
[r] Revised
[W] Withheld to avoid disclosing proprietary data; excluded from "total"

Table 2. Demand for asbestos in the USA
(Thousand tonnes) (US Department of Interior, 1986, 1991)

	1977	1984	1991
Asbestos-cement pipe	115	37	4
Asbestos-cement sheet	27	12	2
Coating and compounds	36	22	1
Flooring products	150	46	-
Friction products	57	48	10
Installation: electrical	4	1	-
Installation: thermal	17	2	-
Packing and gaskets	28	13	3
Paper products	7	2	-
Plastics	8	1	-
Roofing products	70	7	15
Textiles	10	2	-
Other	143	33	1
Total[a]	672	226	34

[a] The totals given are not the exact sums of the values for individual products, owing to independent rounding.

3.2.2 Manufacture of products

Chrysotile use today mainly involves products where it is incorporated into matrices. The asbestos-cement industry is by far the largest user of asbestos fibres world-wide, accounting for some 85% of all use. Asbestos-cement production facilities exist in more than 100 countries and produce 27 to 30 million tonnes annually (Pigg, 1994). Asbestos-cement products contain 10-15% of asbestos, mostly chrysotile, although limited amounts of crocidolite have been used in large diameter, high-pressure pipes.

There are five major asbestos-cement products: (a) corrugated sheets; (b) flat sheets and building boards; (c) slates; (d) moulded goods, including low-pressure pipes; and (e) high-pressure water pipes (Pigg, 1994).

Possible emission sources are: (a) feeding of asbestos fibres into the mix; (b) blending the mix; and (c) cutting or machining end-products. Emissions may vary according to the dust control measures and technology.

Although declining in the North American and Western European markets, asbestos-cement product manufacturing continues to grow in South America, South-East Asia, the eastern Mediterranean region and eastern Europe (Pigg, 1994). Japan, Thailand, Malaysia, Korea and Taiwan imported 430 000 tonnes, well over 30% of world-wide imports in 1989 (Industrial Minerals, 1990). It has been reported that "asbestos use" (the generic term used by the author) in Japan has reached proportions which indicate that it leads the world in consumption of fibres (Frank, 1995).

Other asbestos products consume smaller quantities of chrysotile asbestos. Friction products, gaskets and asbestos paper are among them. Production of shipboard and building insulation, roofing and, particularly, flooring felts and other flooring materials, such as vinyl asbestos tiles, has declined considerably, some of them having disappeared completely from the market place. Friable asbestos materials in building construction have been phased out in many countries due to international recommendations.

Moulded brake linings on disc- and drum-type car brakes are among the chrysotile products that are still manufactured. Woven brake linings and clutch facings for heavy vehicle use are made from high-strength chrysotile yarn and fabric reinforced with wire; this material is dried and impregnated with resin. In the moulding process, the fibres are combined with the resin, which is then thermoset. Final treatment involves curing by baking and grinding to customer specifications.

3.2.3 Use of products

Many chrysotile-containing products have entered global commerce. The nature of the product and local work practices determine dust emissions. Non-friable products and appropriate technological controls greatly reduce fibre release. Manipulation of friable products without controls may release high levels of airborne dust. However, some conditions may produce chrysotile aerosols even with non-friable products, e.g., the use of high-speed power tools without controls.

Concern about the possible exposure of inhabitants of buildings with asbestos-containing materials has led to extensive monitoring (HEI, 1991). In this respect the exposure of custodian and maintenance staff is still being studied (see Chapter 4).

Manufacturing data are not available from individual countries concerning specific chrysotile-containing products.

4. OCCUPATIONAL AND ENVIRONMENTAL EXPOSURE LEVELS

Few recent reports of occupational and environmental exposure levels are available, particularly those that differentiate among the forms of asbestos. Workplace concentrations were very high when monitoring first began (in the 1930s). In countries where controls were implemented, the levels generally reduced considerably with time and continue to decline. In contrast, there is less difference between the early results of measurements in both outdoor and indoor non-occupational environments (1970s) and recent data.

Environmental Health Criteria 53 (IPCS, 1986) reported that 58.5% of samples had fibre concentrations of < 0.5 f/ml and 80.7% < 1.0 f/ml in textile industries in the United Kingdom over the period 1972–1978. Corresponding measurements in France in 1984 were 65.3% with < 0.5 f/ml and 85.4% with < 1.0 f/ml. It also reported 86.5% of samples with < 0.5 f/ml and 95.0% with < 1 f/ml in asbestos-cement industries in the United Kingdom during the period 1972–1978. Corresponding measurements in France in 1984 were 93.5% with < 0.5 f/ml and 97.4% with < 1.0 f/ml. In industries manufacturing friction products, 71.0% of samples had < 0.5 f/ml and 85.5% < 1.0 f/ml in the United Kingdom during 1972–1978, while the corresponding results in France in 1984 were 62.8% with < 0.5 f/ml and 85.0% with < 1.0 f/ml. Typical concentrations (fibres > 5 μm in length) in outdoor air measured in various locations in Austria, Canada, Germany, South Africa and the USA ranged from < 0.0001 to about 0.01 f/ml, concentrations in most samples being less than 0.001 f/ml. Concentrations (fibres > 5 μm in length) measured in various buildings in Canada and Germany ranged from values below the limit of detection to 0.01 f/ml. The highest concentrations were found in buildings with sprayed-on friable asbestos.

4.1 Occupational exposure

This section focuses mainly on exposures found in industries where only commercial chrysotile was used. Emphasis is placed on data obtained directly by the membrane filter method, but, in the case of some older studies, data are conversions from original particle

Occupational and Environmental Exposure Levels

counts. In the latter case, fibre concentrations are subject to the limitations discussed in sections 2.4.1 and 2.4.2.

4.1.1 Mining and milling

Several sets of data have been published concerning the exposure levels of mine and mill workers employed in the production facilities of Thetford Mines and Asbestos, Quebec, Canada. A substantial body of exposure data was collected by using midget impingers and enumerating all dust particles (Gibbs & Lachance, 1972). Table 3 lists mean concentrations of dust in the mills in millions of particles per m^3 (mpcm) and per cubic foot (mpcf) of air during the period 1949 to 1965. The mill with the highest dust concentrations had more than twice the mean values given in Table 3, and that with the lowest concentrations had less than one half.

Table 3. Mean dust concentrations in asbestos mills of Quebec, Canada (from Gibbs & Lachance, 1972)

Concentration	1949	1951	1953	1955	1957	1959	1961	1963	1965
mpcm	2650	1940	1770	1130	1060	570	350	530	180
mpcf	75	55	50	32	30	16	10	15	5

Studies of the relationships between particle counts and fibre concentrations have shown poor correlation (Gibbs & Lachance, 1974; Dagbert, 1976). Gibbs & Lachance (1974) stated that no single conversion factor could be applied to all mines and mills. Assuming a conversion factor of roughly 106 f/ml for each mpcm (3 f/ml for each mpcf), it can be calculated that mean fibre concentrations in the Quebec mills before mid-1955 were well above 150 f/ml (see discussions in section 2.4).

Nicholson et al. (1979) reported fibre concentrations obtained by the membrane filter method in five mines and mills of Thetford Mines, Quebec, Canada during the period October 1973 to October 1975 (Table 4).

Table 4. Asbestos fibre concentrations[a] in five chrysotile mines and mills at Thetford Mines, Quebec, Canada (from Nicholson et al., 1979)

Location		Five mines and mills				
		1	2	3	4	5
General mill air	Number of samples	14	37	5	6	7
	mean	35	12	15	18	9
	range	14–57	7–27	7–27	12–29	5–12
Bagging asbestos	Number of samples	2	6	2	2	
	mean	16	16	9	16	
	range	12–20	10–24	4–13	14–17	
Quality control	Number of samples		2	1	1	
	mean		22	20	9	
	range		21–22	-	-	
Crusher	Number of samples		4			
	mean		26			
	range		8–47			
Dryer	Number of samples		2			
	mean		36			
	range		27–45			
Shops	Number of samples		3			
	mean		10			
	range		6–15			
Non-work location	Number of samples	1	2			
	mean	0.8	1.3			
	range	-	1–1.7			

[a] The concentration of fibres (> 5 µm) is given in f/ml.

In Zimbabwe, Cullen et al. (1991) reported estimates of fibre levels prior to 1980. After 1980, the measured concentrations were below 10 f/ml in all facilities. In India, the concentrations measured in four mills in 1989 by Mukherjee et al. (1992) are presented in Table 5.

Table 5. Average personal sample fibre concentrations in four mills in India (from Mukherjee et al., 1992)

Process	Fibre concentration (f/ml)	
	Average	Range
Jaw crusher	1.7	1.3–2.1
Pulverizer	8.9	2.3–15.4
Lime mixer	2.6	2.5–2.6
Huller	12.7	8.9–16.4
Primary concentric screen	12.9	1.8–25.8
Decorticator	8.8	1.3–18.4

Parsons et al. (1986) reported that the concentrations in refining and bagging areas in a Newfoundland mill were generally less than 0.5 f/ml, but concentrations in the screening area ranged up to 13.9 f/ml.

Average concentrations of asbestos fibres (length > 5 μm) in the Quebec mining industry during the period 1973–1993 are presented in Fig. 1. The average concentrations in Quebec chrysotile mining towns are shown in Fig. 2.

4.1.2 Textile production

Nine textile plants in the USA were studied in 1964 and 1965 by Lynch & Ayer (1966). The results of the membrane filter analysis are presented in Table 6. The presence of small amounts of amosite or crocidolite fibres cannot be excluded due to the non-specificity of the assay instrument (PCOM).

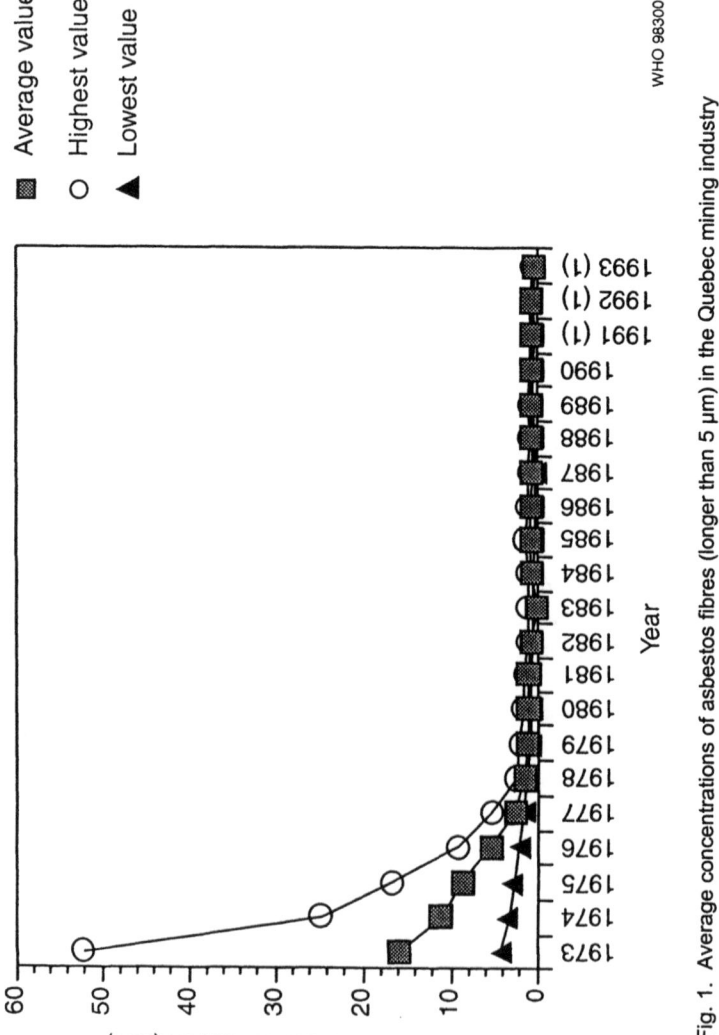

Fig. 1. Average concentrations of asbestos fibres (longer than 5 μm) in the Quebec mining industry (Lebel, 1995a,b)

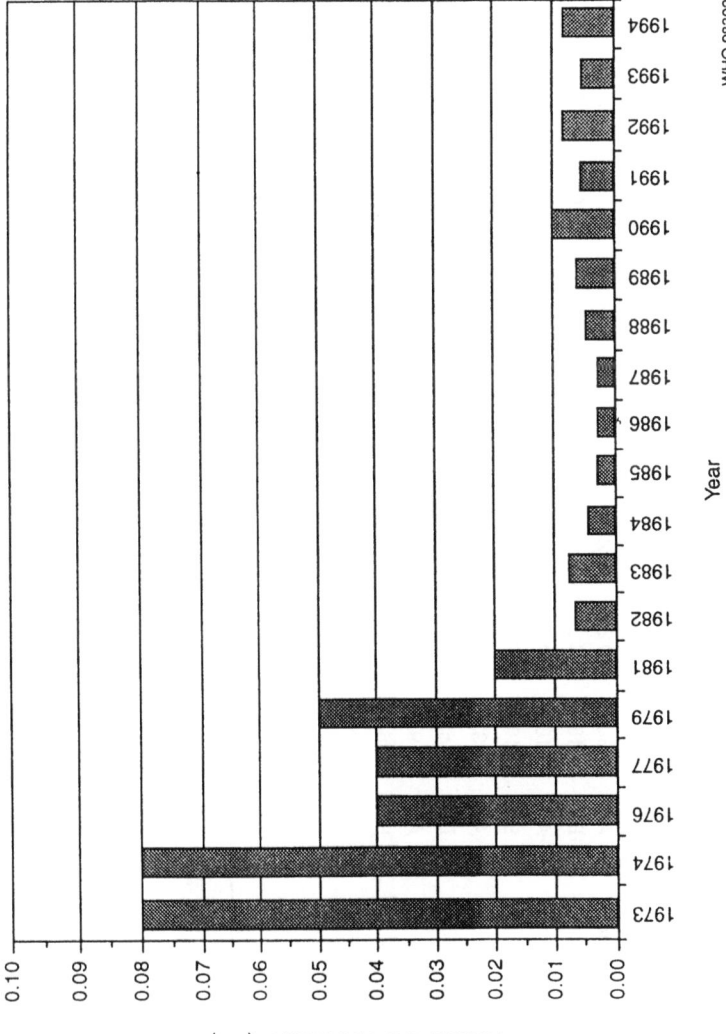

Fig. 2. Asbestos fibre concentrations in Quebec chrysotile mining towns (Lebel, 1995a,b)

Table 6. Mean dust concentrations (f/ml) by plant and operation in nine textile plants in the USA during the period 1964/1965 (from Lynch & Ayer, 1966)

Operation	Fibres[a]	Textile plants								
		1	2	3	4	5	6	7	8	9
Fibre preparation	A	38.1	12.3	23.3	34.0	-	8.1	7.6	35.5	11.8
	B	15.0	10.0	13.3	18.3	-	3.0	4.5	17.0	2.6
Carding	A	18.1	13.6	20.6	32.9	-	6.0	17.2	28.2	8.3
	B	10.2	9.21	3.3	15.2	-	3.5	8.1	13.4	2.0
Spinning	A	9.6	4.1	20.2	29.8	-	5.1	24.8	20.8	7.4
	B	6.6	3.2	18.9	15.7	-	3.5	10.8	10.5	1.8
Twisting	A	9.3	6.9	15.8	51.4	-	4.8	25.9	16.7	3.1
	B	6.4	5.2	7.5	22.4	-	3.3	12.9	7.2	1.1
Winding	A	11.7	4.4	9.6	28.6	-	4.5	25.7	7.9	3.6
	B	7.5	3.9	8.9	17.5	-	3.2	11.7	2.7	1.3
Weaving	A	7.7	7.0	2.9	33.8	4.5	2.9	9.5	8.1	2.9
	B	4.8	3.1	2.3	17.8	3.9	2.2	5.7	3.0	1.5

[a] A = total fibres, B = fibres longer than 5 µm

The exposure estimates (1930–1975) in an extensively studied textile plant in South Carolina, USA, in which chrysotile was the predominant fibre used, are presented in Table 7 (Dement et al., 1983a).

Table 7. Exposure estimates in a chrysotile textile plant (1930-1975) (estimated mean exposure to fibres longer than 5 μm in f/ml)[a]

Operation	Without controls	With controls
Fibre preparation	26.2–78.0	5.8–17.2
Carding	10.8–22.1	4.3–9.0
Spinning	4.8–8.2	4.8–6.7
Twisting	24.6–36.0	5.4–7.9
Winding	4.1–20.9	4.1–8.4
Weaving	5.3–30.6	1.4–8.2

[a] From: Dement et al. (1983a)

Application of controls in the dusty processes at the South Carolina plant led to significant reduction of exposure. Currently available control technology allows much lower levels to be attained.

Table 8 shows a summary of exposure classifications in an English textile plant in the period 1951–1974 (Peto et al., 1985). The early particle count data in this report were based on fibre collection with a thermal precipitator. The conversion factor used, therefore, reflects only a precipitator-membrane filter relationship. Comments on the validity of such conversions have been discussed by Walton (1982).

Kimura (1987) reported geometric mean concentrations of 2.6–12.8 f/ml in the period 1970–1975 and 0.1–0.2 f/ml in the period 1984–1986 in asbestos spinning in Japan.

Table 8. Mean concentrations of airborne asbestos fibres in a textile plant[a]

Period	Very high	High	Medium	Low
1951–1955[b]	unloading, stacking 28 f/ml	roving, spinning, carding 14 f/ml	doubling, rope spinning 8 f/ml	other areas 4.5 f/ml
1956–1960[b]	unloading, stacking 28 f/ml	carding 16 f/ml	roving, spinning, mixing 9 f/ml	other areas 4.5 f/ml
1961–1965	unloading, stacking 20 f/ml	carding 15 f/ml	carding, roving, winding, beaming 7.5 f/ml	other areas 2.5 f/ml
1966–1970	unloading, stacking 20 f/ml	carding 15 f/ml	carding, roving, rope cards 7.5 f/ml	other areas 2.5 f/ml
1971–1974	none	none	carding, roving 7.5 f/ml	other areas 2.5 f/ml

[a] Peto et al. (1985)
[b] Results of particle measurements were converted to fibre concentrations using the relationship 35 p/ml = 1 f/ml

4.1.3 Asbestos-cement

As mentioned in section 3.2.2, the principal use of chrysotile in the world today is in asbestos-cement products. In the production of asbestos-cement pipes, some crocidolite is still used with chrysotile in certain plants.

Table 9 summarizes the results of the analysis of personal samples, collected in the late 1970s when reportedly only chrysotile was used, in an asbestos-cement facility in the USA (Hammad et al., 1979). In 80% of the samples the concentrations were less than 2 f/ml, and in about 60% they were less than 0.5 f/ml.

Table 9. Chrysotile fibre concentrations (fibres longer than 5 µm) in selected dust zones of an asbestos-cement production facility[a]

Location	Number of samples	Fibre concentration (f/ml) range	mean
Regrinding	4	0.44–1.2	0.86
Mixing	9	0.51–8.9	2.8
Forming	20	0.12–5.0	0.52
Siding and shingle finishing	14	0.14–4.9	0.68
Panel finishing	11	0.33–12.0	2.8
Flat and corrugated finishing	12	0.33–8.0	2.6
Warehouse	5	0.13–2.5	0.63
Maintenance	7	0.20–2.7	0.58

[a] From: Hammad et al. (1979)

Exposure estimates in a Canadian plant (Finkelstein, 1983) for the years 1949, 1969 and 1979 were 40, 20 and 0.2 f/ml, respectively, for willow operators, 16, 8 and 0.5 f/ml for forming machine operators, and 8, 4 and 0.3 f/ml for lathe operators. In Japan, Kimura (1987) reported geometric mean concentrations in bag opening and mixing of 4.5–9.5 f/ml in 1970–1975 and 0.03–1.6 f/ml in 1984–1986, whilst in cement cutting and grinding the mean concentrations were 2.5–3.5 f/ml in 1970–1975 and 0.17–0.57 in 1984–1986. Albin et al. (1990) reported fibre concentrations, based on estimates, in a Swedish asbestos-cement plant of 1.5–6.3 f/ml during 1956. Later, based on direct measurements, values were 0.3–5.0 f/ml in 1969 and 0.9–1.7 f/ml in 1975. Higashi et al. (1994) reported geometric average concentrations of 0.05–0.45 f/ml measured in area samples and 0.05–0.78 f/ml in personal samples of an asbestos-cement plant.

Few data are available in the open literature on exposures encountered during installation of asbestos-cement products. It would be expected that cutting, sanding, drilling or otherwise abrading asbestos-cement without efficient ventilation controls would give rise to high exposures (Nicholson, 1978).

Weiner et al. (1994) reported concentrations in a South African workshop in which chrysotile asbestos-cement sheets were cut into components for insulation. The sheets were cut manually, sanded and subsequently assembled. Initial sampling showed personal sample mean concentrations of 1.9 f/ml for assembling, 5.7 f/ml for sweeping, 8.6 f/ml for drilling and 27.5 f/ml for sanding. After improvements and clean-up of the work environment, the concentrations were 0.5–1.7 f/ml.

Nicholson (1978) reported concentrations of 0.33–1.47 f/ml in a room during and after sawing and hammering of an asbestos-cement panel.

4.1.4 Friction products

Skidmore & Dufficy (1983), based on simulated past conditions (Table 10), and McDonald et al. (1984) reported data on workplace exposures during friction product manufacturing.

McDonald et al. (1984) reported that in the 1930s estimated average dust levels were 35-180 mpcm (1-5 mpcf) in 67% of analysed locations, while in the 1960s average dust levels were below 7 mpcm (0.2 mpcf) at 38% of locations and below 18 mpcm (0.5 mpcf) at 67% of locations in which measurements were obtained.

Table 10. Average concentrations of chrysotile fibres (f/ml) longer > 5 μm from woven asbestos products during various periods

	Pre-1931	1932-1950	1951-1969	1970-1979
Storage/distribution	>20	2–5	2–5	0.5–1
Preparation	>20	0–20	2–5	1–2
Impregnation/forming	>20	2–5	1–2	0.5–1
Grinding	>20	5–10	2–5	0.5–1
Drilling, boring	>20	2–5	1–2	1–2
Inspection	>20	2–5	1–2	0.5–1
Packing	>20	1–2	0.5–1	<0.5
Office/laboratory	10–20	<0.5	<0.5	<0.5

*Skidmore & Dufficy (1983)

Kimura (1987) reported geometric mean fibre concentrations of 10.2–35.5 f/ml in 1970–1975, and 0.24–5.5 f/ml in 1984–1986 in spinning and grinding of friction products in Japan.

A considerable number of reports have included airborne asbestos concentrations during maintenance and replacement of vehicle brakes. In the early period, poor or no engineering control measures were utilized, resulting in high total dust exposure. This was particularly so during grinding of brakes and compressed air blowing off dust, both operations of very short duration. Significantly lower levels were measured when engineering controls were introduced.

An overview of air concentrations measured during maintenance and replacement of asbestos-containing vehicle brakes is presented in Table 11.

4.1.5 Exposure of building maintenance personnel

The subject of asbestos exposure of maintenance personnel in buildings has been raised recently and particularly by US OSHA (1994).

Table 11. Asbestos air concentrations measured during maintenance and replacement of vehicle brakes

Mean concentration (f/ml)	Comment	Reference
3.8[a]	grinding truck brakes	Lorimer et al., 1976
15.9[a]	blowing off	Lorimer et al., 1976
3.8[a]	grinding	Rohl et al., 1976
16.0[a]	blowing off	Rohl et al., 1976
2.5[a]	dry brushing	Rohl et al., 1976
>1[a]	17 of 19 operations	Menichini & Marconi, 1982
>2[a]	11 of 19 operations	Menichini & Marconi, 1982
0.09[b]	fibres longer than 5 µm	Jahn et al., 1985
6.2[a]	blowing off, grinding	Jahn et al., 1985
0.03[b]	fibres longer than 5 µm	Elliehausen, 1985
0.06[b]		Ruhe & Lipscomb, 1985
<0.5	TWA	Cheng & O'Kelly, 1986
0.13	maximum	Cheng & O'Kelly, 1986
4–5[a]	fibres longer than 5 µm, blowing off, grinding	Rodelsperger et al., 1986
5–10[a]	fibres longer than 5 µm, blowing off, grinding, trucks	Rodelsperger et al., 1986
<0.05[b]		Kauppinen & Korhonen, 1987
0.01–0.2[b]	trucks and buses	Kauppinen & Korhonen, 1987

Table 11 (contd).

> 1[a]	blowing off	Kauppinen & Korhonen, 1987
< 0.004		Sheehy et al., 1987
< 0.004[b]		Godbey et al., 1987
0.09–0.12		Van Wagenen, 1987
0.046[b]		Cooper et al., 1988
0.03[b]	TWA < 0.002 f/ml	Moore, 1988

[a] These results are mean personal samples obtained by PCOM; fibres $\geq$ 5 µm; these represent episodic releases and not time-weighted averages; operation specific.
[b] Mean personal air samples (8-h time-weighted average)

Price et al. (1992) estimated the time-weighted averages (TWAs), of asbestos exposures experienced by maintenance personnel, on the basis of 1227 air samples. The TWAs, obtained by PCOM, were 0.009 f/ml for telecommunication switch work, 0.037 f/ml for above-ceiling maintenance work, and 0.51 f/ml for work in utility spaces. Median concentrations ranged from 0.01 to 0.02 f/ml.

The Health Effects Institute (1991) evaluated an operation and maintenance programme in a hospital on the basis of 394 air samples obtained during 106 on-site activities. The mean asbestos concentration (PCOM) was about 0.11 f/ml for personal samples and about 0.012 f/ml for area samples. Eight-hour TWA concentrations showed that 99% of the personal samples were below 0.2 f/ml, and 95% were below 0.1 f/ml.

Corn et al. (1994) evaluated exposures of building maintenance personnel on the basis of about 500 personal samples collected during maintenance work. However, the building personnel were being monitored during an asbestos "operations and management" programme, so that these values may reflect special work practices and environment conditions. Typical personal exposures are presented in Table 12.

Table 12. Personal asbestos exposures of building maintenance personnel (fibres longer than 5 μm)[a]

Activity	Concentration during work (f/ml)	8-h TWA
Electrical/plumbing work	0–0.035	0.0149
Cable running	0.001–0.228	0.0167
HVAC work	0–0.077	0.0023

[a] From: Corn (1994)

Published data for custodial workers, as they exist, reflect unusual circumstances. Sawyer (1977) studied fibre release from a friable chrysotile-containing surface formulation during routine custodial activities performed in the Yale Art and Architecture Building. The fibre levels, determined by PCOM, ranged from 1.6 f/ml, obtained during sweeping, to 15.5 f/ml, obtained during dusting of library books. These values were obtained as short-term episodes. Most other values, presented as 8-h TWAs, were about two orders of magnitude lower (HEI, 1991).

4.1.6 Various industries

Higashi et al. (1994) reported the results of their environmental evaluations at 510 workplaces in 1985 (roofing materials, asbestos-cement sheets, friction materials, construction materials) and 430 workplaces in 1992. The percentage of workplaces in which exposure concentrations were less than 0.3 f/ml was 70% in 1985 and 98% in 1992. All concentrations in a modernized asbestos-cement plant were less than 0.1 f/ml.

Rickards (1991, 1994) reported the results of the measurement of asbestos fibre concentrations covering exposures of over 39 900 workers in 27 countries in 1989 and over 26 500 workers in 28 countries in 1991 and 1992. His modified results are presented in Table 13. The 1993 data, by industry sector, is shown in Fig. 3 (AIA, 1995). Kogevinas et al. (1994) summarized exposure data obtained from chrysotile-exposed workers in 11 countries. The exposure levels ranged considerably, reflecting industry and other factors.

Table 13. Percentages of over 26 500 workers in 28 countries exposed to various asbestos fibre concentrations in the workplace (members of Asbestos International Association)[a]

	Asbestos fibre concentration (f/ml)			
	< 0.5	0.5-1	1-2	> 2
Percentage of workers				
1989	83.5	11.1	4.5	0.9
1991	84.4	9.4	4.2	2.1
1992	89.1	6.3	3.9	0.8

[a] Rickards (1991, 1994)

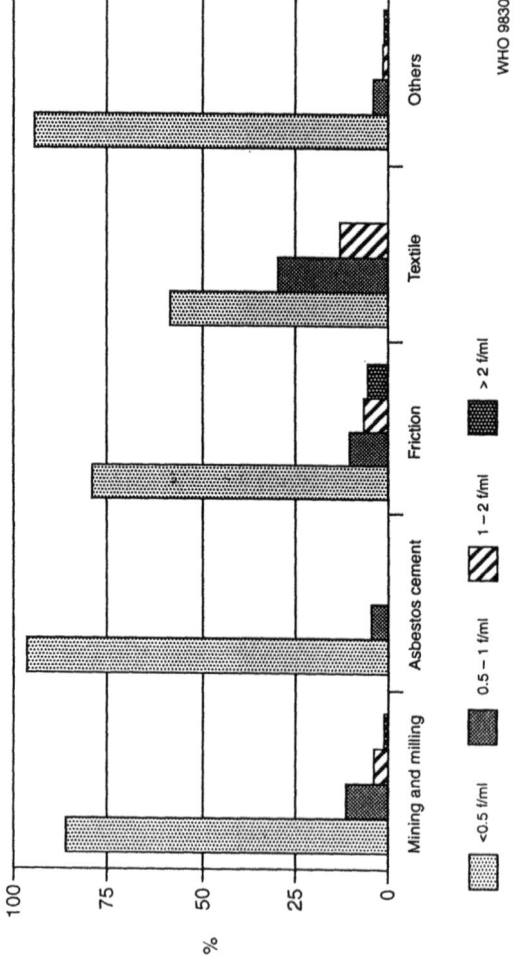

Fig. 3. Percentages of workers exposed to various asbestos fibre concentrations in 1993 (AIA, 1995)

Fei & Huang (1989) reported fibre concentrations in an asbestos paper factory utilizing chrysotile in the Sichuan Province of west China. The concentration of 135 fibre measurements ranged between 0.6 f/ml and 55.1 f/ml, the latter value being the average of 6 assays in a pulp-reducing area.

4.2 Non-occupational exposure

4.2.1 Ambient air

There are some data concerning fibre levels in the air close to chrysotile mines. Baloyi (1989) found fibre levels around the Shabani Mine (Zimbabwe) to range from below the limit of detection of the method (< 0.01 f/ml) to 0.02 f/ml of air, assayed by PCOM.

Asbestos concentrations in the outdoor air have been measured in many studies. Chrysotile is the predominant fibre found. Concentrations measured at various locations in Austria, Canada, Germany, South Africa and the USA were reported in Environmental Health Criteria 53 (IPCS, 1986; Table 14). Typical concentrations of fibres longer than 5 µm ranged from less than 0.0001 f/ml to about 0.01 f/ml, most samples having concentrations less than 0.001 f/ml. Results of some more recent studies are presented in Table 14. Almost all analyses were made by TEM. A review of available data was given in HEI (1991).

Corn (1994) estimated that outdoor air concentrations, expressed as PCOM equivalent fibres (longer than 5 µm), in remote locations in the USA are generally less than 0.0005 f/ml, in urban areas they are up to 0.002 f/ml, and in suburban locations they are considerably lower.

4.2.2 Indoor air

Concentrations measured in various buildings in Canada and Germany were presented in Environmental Health Criteria 53 (IPCS, 1986, Table 12). Concentration of fibres longer than 5 µm ranged from below the detectable level of the method to 0.01 f/ml. The highest concentrations were found in buildings with sprayed-on asbestos.

Table 14. Asbestos fibre concentrations in outdoor air
(f/ml PCOM equivalent fibres[a] - TEM)

Environment	Median	Mean	Range[f]	Reference
Rural				
Japan	0.0218		0.007–0.047	Kohyama, 1989
Urban				
Switzerland		<0.0004[b]		Litistorf et al., 1985
USA	0.0003[c]		ND–0.008	Chesson et al., 1985
Canada	0.0007		0.0006–0.0009	Sebastien et al., 1986a
USA		0.00005[c]		Tuckfield et al., 1988
Canada	0.0001[b]		ND–0.003	Nicholson, 1988
Japan		0.0198[e]	<0.004–0.111	Kohyama, 1989
England		0.00016[b]	ND–0.00016	Jaffrey, 1988
England		0.0004[b]		Jaffrey, 1990
Slovak Republic		0.002[d]	0.001–0.02	Juck et al., 1991
Italy			0.0001–0.012	Chiappino et al., 1993

[a] PCOM equivalent fibre: >5 μm long; ≥ 0.25 μm wide; aspect ratio ≥ 3:1
[b] total structures >5 μm
[c] PCOM analysis
[d] near to an asbestos-cement plant
[e] residential area
[f] ND - not detected

The results of some more recent studies are presented in Table 15.

Table 15. Asbestos fibre concentrations (f/ml) in buildings
(fibres longer than 5 μm)

Site[a]	Mean[b]	Range[b]	Reference
Canada			
High-rise office	0.0034	0.0002–0.0065	Chatfield, 1986
Schools	0.0006	ND–0.0014	Chatfield, 1986
United Kingdom			
Buildings with ACM		ND–0.0017	Burdett & Jaffrey, 1986
Buildings without ACM		ND–0.0007	Burdett & Jaffrey, 1986

Table 15 (contd).

Site[a]	Mean[b]	Range[b]	Reference
United Kingdom (contd)			
Residences with ACM	0.0003	ND–0.0025	Gazzi & Crockford, 1987
Residences without ACM	ND	ND	Gazzi & Crockford, 1987
USA			
Residences with ACM	0.0001	ND–0.002	CPSC, 1987
Buildings with ACM	0.00005	ND–0.00056	Hatfield et al., 1988; Crump & Farrar, 1989; Chesson et al., 1990
Buildings without ACM	ND	ND	Hatfield et al., 1988; Crump & Farrar, 1989; Chesson et al., 1990
Schools	0.00024	ND–0.0023	Corn et al., 1991
Schools with ACM	0.0002	ND–0.0016	McCrone, 1991
Slovak Republic			
Buildings	0.0045	0.00085–0.024	Juck et al., 1991
Belgium			
Public buildings		0.0045–0.0061	Minne et al., 1991

[a] ACM = asbestos-containing material
[b] ND = not detected

The average airborne fibre concentrations in outdoor air, 71 schools and 49 public buildings in the USA are presented in Table 16.

Table 16. Mean concentrations of asbestos fibres longer than 5 µm[a]

	Sample size	Mean concentration (f/ml)
Outdoor air	48	0.00039
Schools	71	0.00024
Public buildings (no ACM)	6	0.00099
Public buildings (with ACM in good condition)	6	0.00059
Public buildings (with damaged ACM)	37	0.00073

[a] Modified from Mossman et al. (1990)

Corn (1994) estimated an average level of PCOM equivalent fibres (> 0.2 μm width) of 0.00017 f/ml in 71 schools in the USA. Five per cent of the school indoor concentrations exceeded 0.0014 f/ml, the highest value being 0.0023 f/ml.

Lee et al. (1992) found that only 0.67% of chrysotile fibres in indoor air are longer than 5 μm.

5. UPTAKE, CLEARANCE, RETENTION AND TRANSLOCATION

5.1 Inhalation

5.1.1 *General principles*

Factors affecting the inhalation, deposition, clearance and translocation of asbestos and other fibres were discussed in Environmental Health Criteria monographs 53 (IPCS, 1986), 77 (IPCS, 1988) and 151 (IPCS, 1993). The main principles are summarized in this subsection.

It is considered that the potential respiratory health effects related to exposure to fibre aerosols are a function of the internal dose to the target tissue, which is determined by airborne concentrations, patterns of exposure, fibre shape, diameter and length (which affect lung deposition and clearance) and biopersistence. The potential responses to fibres, once they are deposited in the lungs, are a function of their individual characteristics.

Because of the tendency of fibres to align parallel to the direction of airflow, the deposition of fibrous particles in the respiratory tract is largely a function of fibre length. In addition, the shape of the fibres as well as their electrostatic charge may have an effect on deposition (Davis et al., 1988). Fibres of various shapes are more likely than spherical particles to be deposited by interception, mainly at bifurcations.

Since most of the data on deposition have been obtained in studies on rodents, it is important to consider comparative differences between rats and humans in this respect; these differences are best evaluated on the basis of the aerodynamic diameter. The ratio of fibre diameter to aerodynamic diameter is approximately 1:3. Thus, a fibre measured microscopically to have a diameter of 1 µm would have a corresponding aerodynamic diameter of approximately 3 µm. A comparative review of the regional deposition of particles in humans and rodents (rats and hamsters) has been presented by US EPA (1980). The relative distribution between the tracheobronchial and pulmonary regions of the lung in rodents follows a pattern similar to human regional deposition during nose breathing for insoluble particles with a mass median aerodynamic diameter of less than 3 µm. Fig. 4 and 5 illustrate these comparative differences. As can be seen, particularly for pulmonary deposition of particles, the percentage deposition in rodents is considerably less, even within the overlapping region of respiratory tract deposition, than in humans. These data indicate that, although particles with an aerodynamic diameter of 5 µm or more may have significant deposition efficiencies in man, the same particles will have extremely small deposition efficiencies in the rodent.

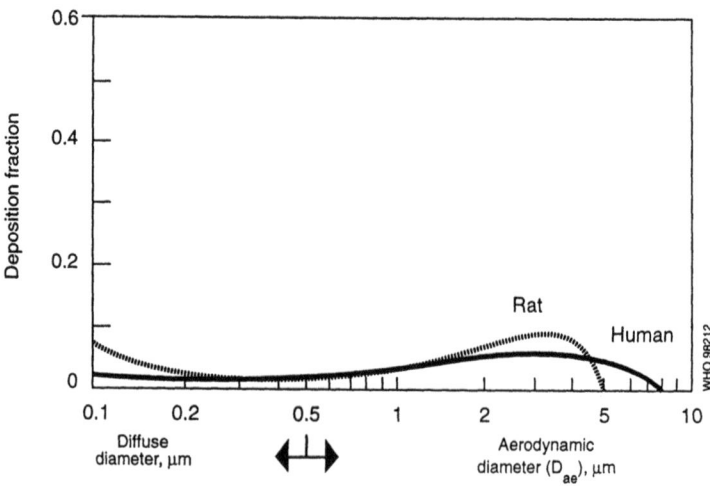

Fig. 4. Tracheobronchial deposition of inhaled monodisperse aerosols in humans and rats (US EPA, 1980)

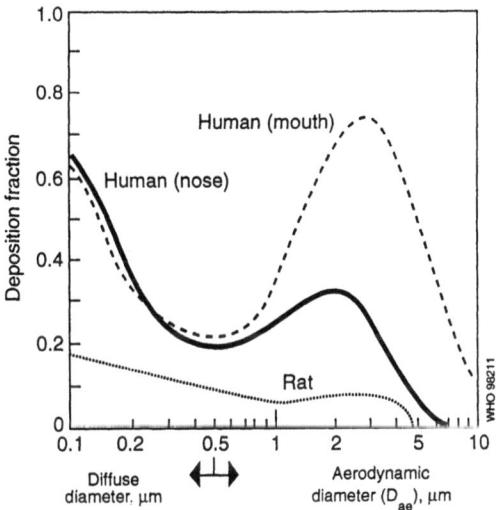

Fig. 5. Pulmonary deposition of inhaled monodisperse aerosols in man and rat (US EPA, 1980)

In the nasopharyngeal and tracheobronchial regions, fibres are generally cleared fairly rapidly via mucociliary clearance, whereas fibres deposited in the alveolar space appear to be cleared more slowly, primarily by phagocytosis and to a lesser extent via translocation and by dissolution. Translocation refers to the movement of the intact fibre after initial deposition at foci in the alveolar ducts and on the ciliated epithelium at the terminal bronchioles. These fibres may be translocated via ciliated mucous movement up the bronchial tree and removed from the lung, or may be moved through the epithelium with subsequent migration to interstitial storage sites or along lymphatic drainage pathways or transport to pleural regions. Fibres short enough to be fully ingested are thought to be removed mainly through phagocytosis by macrophages, whereas longer fibres may be partially cleared at a slower rate either by translocation to interstitial sites, breakage or by dissolution. A higher proportion of longer fibres is, therefore, retained in the lung.

5.1.2 Fibre deposition

The deposition of chrysotile asbestos in the peripheral lung airways of rats exposed *in vivo* for 1 h to 4.3 mg respirable chrysotile/m^3 was studied by Brody et al. (1981). In rats killed immediately after exposure, chrysotile fibres were rarely seen by scanning electron microscopy in alveolar spaces or on alveolar duct surfaces, except at alveolar duct bifurcations. Most were less than 10 µm in length and 0.4 µm in diameter, indicating that longer fibres present in the dust cloud had been deposited in the upper airways. Concentrations were relatively high at bifurcations nearest the terminal bronchioles, and lower at the bifurcations of more distal ducts. In rats killed after 5 h the patterns were similar, but the concentrations were reduced. The relative importance of interception, impaction, diffusion and sedimentation on the deposition pattern of chrysotile fibres was considered by Brody & Roe (1983) who concluded that the high deposition observed at alveolar duct bifurcations of rats can be attributed to the high breathing frequency and small airway size of these rodents. They pointed out that the enhanced deposition at alveolar duct bifurcations observed in the rat may not occur in all species.

Coin et al. (1992) examined the patterns of deposition and retention of chrysotile asbestos in the central and peripheral regions of the rat lung in the first month following a single 3-h inhalation exposure. They found that pulmonary deposition did not differ between peripheral and central regions.

Pinkerton & Yu (1988) exposed rats to airborne chrysotile fibres for 7 h/day, 5 days/week for 12 months, and investigated the numbers and lengths of chrysotile fibres found in anatomically distinct regions of the lung parenchyma. The fibre concentration was greatest in the dorsal region and least in the costolateral and caudal regions, in agreement with calculations based on the deposition model for rat lung of Asgharian & Yu (1988). With the exception of the dorsal region, parenchymal changes correlated well with the fibre concentration. There were differences in the length distributions of fibres in the various regions, fibres in the dorsal region having the greatest proportion of fibres longer than 10 µm. The proportion of fibres longer than 20 µm was greatest in the cranial and lateral regions.

5.1.3 Fibre clearance and retention

5.1.3.1 Fibre clearance and retention in humans

Available data obtained from lung burden studies show that chrysotile fibres deposited in the lung are cleared more rapidly than tremolite fibres, so that the tremolite/chrysotile ratio increases with time after exposure. It has been shown by Sebastien et al. (1989) and Churg et al. (1993) that on average about 75% of the fibres in the lungs of long-term chrysotile miners and millers from the Thetford Mines region of Quebec were tremolite and only about 25% chrysotile, despite the fact that tremolite accounted for only a few percent of the fibres in the chrysotile ambient dust (Sebastien et al., 1986a). Rowlands et al. (1982) found similar quantities of tremolite fibres, compared with chrysotile, in the lung samples of Quebec miners and millers. Limitations of retention data in lungs with respect to chrysotile exposure have been discussed in a review by Case et al. (1994).

5.1.3.2 Fibre clearance and retention in laboratory animals

Several studies on laboratory animals, mainly rats, have investigated the lung clearance of chrysotile as measured by changes in the lung retention of fibres following acute, short-term and long-term inhalation or single dose via intratracheal exposure. Results of these studies are summarized in Table 17.

Morgan et al. (1977) used a radiotracer technique to study the lung clearance of chrysotile A, chrysotile B, amosite, crocidolite and anthophyllite asbestos following short nose-only inhalation exposures (3 h). There was a rapid decline in fibre lung content followed by a slow phase. The initial decline was assumed to represent mucocilliary clearance of fibres deposited in the smaller conducting airways, and the slow phase to alveolar clearance. Half-times of alveolar clearance, measured over a period of several months following exposure, were in the range of 60–90 days. No significant difference was observed between amphibole and chrysotile asbestos.

Table 17. Studies of chrysotile clearance in experimental animals

Species	Number of animals	Protocol[a]	Results[a]	Reference
Rats (SPF Wistar)	total of 1013 rats: group size of 19-58	Groups exposed to 9.7–14.7 mg/m^3 of UICC amos, anthophyl, croc, chrys A & chrys B for periods of 1 day, 3,6,12 or 24 months.	Linear increase in lung burden of amphiboles with time. Much less chrys found in lung and no clear increase with dose.	Wagner et al., 1974
Rats (Albino male)	total of 56 rats: group size of 8	Groups exposed nose-only to neutron-activated UICC amos, anthophyl, croc, chrys A & chrys B for 1 h. Deposition measured radiometrically.	Half-time clearance about 3 months. Fibres translocated to subpleural sites.	Morgan et al., 1977
Rats (SPF Wistar AF/HAN strain)	not specified	Groups exposed to 1, 5 and 10 mg/m^3 of UICC amos, croc and chrys A 7 h/day, 5 days/week for 6 weeks. Asbestos in lung measured by ashing and infrared spectrophotometry.	Deposition rate of chrys 25% of that of amphiboles but clearance rate independent of fibre type.	Middleton et al., 1979
Rats (CD-1 strain male)	total of 15 rats: group size of 3	Groups exposed nose-only to 4.3 mg/m^3 chrys for 1 h. Distribution of fibres in lung measured by SEM and TEM at times from 1 h to 8 days.	Most fibres deposited at bifurcations of alveolar ducts. Fibres taken up by Type 1 epithelial cells.	Brody et al., 1981
Rats (Wistar female)	unspecified	Groups instilled intratracheally with 2 mg UICC chrys A. Rats killed at 1 day, 1, 6, 12, 18 and 24 months after instillation. Fibre numbers and composition determined after low-temperature ashing of lung using TEM and ATEM.	Number of chrys fibres increased with time and also their mean length.	Bellmann et al., 1987

Table 17 (contd).

Guinea-pigs (Hartley strain female)	total of 18 animals	Animals instilled intratracheally with a mixture of UICC chrys B and amos. Sub-groups of 6 animals killed at 1 day, 1 week and 1 month after administration. Fibre concentration in lung tissue determined using hypochlorite digests of tissue with TEM and EDXA.	Chrys fibre concentration declined more rapidly than that of amos. Concentration ratio declined from 8:1 to 2:1.	Churg et al., 1989
Rats (SPF Sprague-Dawley male)	total of 23 animals	Animals exposed to 10 mg/m³ chrys for 3 h. Subgroups were killed immediately after exposure and after 1, 8, 15 and 29 days. Peripheral and central regions of the left lung digested and fibres characterized by SEM.	Deposition similar in central and peripheral regions. Average diameter of fibres decreased with time and length increased.	Coin et al., 1994
Rats (Fischer 344 male)	not specified	Exposures nose-only to 10–15 mg/m³. Chrys: 7 h/day, 5 days/week for 6 weeks Croc: 6 h/day, 5 days/week for 90 days Animals sacrificed 90 days after exposure.	In lungs of chrys- and croc-exposed rats longer and narrower fibres than in airborne dust. 90 days post-exposure 95% clearance of chrys, no clearance of croc (by fibre numbers).	Abraham et al., 1988
Rats (Sprague-Dawley male)	total of 48 rats: group size of 8	Groups exposed to 5 mg/m³ UICC Canadian chrys for 5 h. Subgroups killed at the end of exposure and after 1, 7, 28 and 90 days. TEM analysis of fibres in lung and BAL.	Progressive increase in mean length, decrease in mean diameter of fibres in lungs. Decrease in mean length and diameter in BAL.	Kauffer et al., 1987

Table 17 (contd).

Species	Number of animals	Protocol[a]	Results[a]	Reference
Hamsters (Syrian golden, sex not specified)	not specified	Animals instilled with one intratracheal dose of 1 mg UICC Canadian chrys or amos in 0.1 ml saline, killed at 4 and 56 weeks, and 2 years (chrys), 2 years (amos). SEM analysis with EDXA.	Ratio of short chrys fibres (<5 µm) decreased from initially 30% to 13% in the lung; 2 years after instillation increased again to 56% (diameter < 0.05 µm). Short amos fibres (< 5 µm) decreased from 41% initially to 4% after 2 years.	Kimizuka et al., 1987
Rats (Barrier derived Fischer 344)	not specified	Rats instilled intratracheally with chrys, croc and erionite at weekly intervals for 21 weeks. Instilled dose of chrys 32 mg. Rats killed at 1 h, 1 day, 1, 4, 8, 12 and 24 months following final instillation. Fibres recovered from lung by low-temperature ashing and analysed by TEM.	Apparent increase in number of chrys fibres between 1 and 10 days followed by gradual decline.	Coffin et al., 1992

Table 17 (contd).

| Rats (SPF Wistar AF/HAN strain male) | not specified | Rats exposed to 10 mg/m³ UICC chrys A for 7 h/day, 5 days/week for up to 18 months. Groups removed from exposure after exposures of 1 day, 4, 13, 26, 52, 65 and 95 weeks, and subgroups killed at 3 and 38 days after removal. Numbers and dimensions of fibres recovered from lung measured by SEM. Fibres with dia > 0.3 µm analysed by EDXA. | Splitting chrys fibres lead to increasing number of long thin fibres with time; after 150 days of exposure lung burden no longer increased. | Jones et al., 1994 |

[a] amos = amosite; croc = crocidolite; chrys = chrysotile; anthophyl = anthophyllite.

Middleton et al. (1979), using UICC samples, exposed rats via inhalation over a 6-week period to concentrations of 1, 5 and 10 mg/m^3 and then estimated the amount of asbestos in lung by infrared spectrophotometry after lung ashing. The fractional deposition of chrysotile was lower than for amosite and crocidolite, but the alveolar clearance rates of chrysotile and amphibole fibres were similar. The lower deposition rate of chrysotile was believed to be related to differences in airborne asbestos concentration during exposure and to the curly nature of chrysotile fibres.

In contrast, Abraham et al. (1988) found that the alveolar clearance of chrysotile was faster than that of crocidolite. In their study, rats were exposed by inhalation to 10–15 mg/m^3 of either chrysotile (6 weeks) or crocidolite (90 days). At the end of exposure, lung fibre concentrations and size distributions were similar for both types of fibres. However, during the subsequent 90 days, 95% of chrysotile (by fibre number) was removed, whereas there was no measurable clearance of crocidolite. Similar findings were reported by Bérubé et al. (1996). The fibre retention of chrysotile in the rat lung after 5 and 20 days of inhalation exposure to 8 mg/m^3 was considerably lower than the fibre lung retention of crocidolite asbestos.

Wagner & Skidmore (1965), in a 6-week inhalation exposure study on rats using about 30 mg/m^3, reported that, over a period of 2 months, the rate of clearance for chrysotile was higher by a factor of 3 than that for amosite or crocidolite. In addition, the retention of chrysotile, as measured a few days after the end of the 6-week exposure period, was only about one third that of the amphiboles.

In a subsequent study by the same group (Wagner et al., 1974), it was found that, while the lung burden of amphibole fibres increased steadily with time, that of chrysotile appeared to reach a plateau after 3 months of exposure and at a much lower level compared to the simultaneous amphibole level. The difference was attributed to the enhanced clearance rate of chrysotile. This difference in the lung clearance of chrysotile and amphibole fibres has been confirmed by several studies (Davies et al., 1978, 1986a; Davis & Jones, 1988) with amphibole levels at the end of a one-year inhalation period in rats being approximately 10 times those of chrysotile administered at the same mass dose. In their inhalation study of the retention of UICC chrysotile fibres in rat lung (10 mg/m^3, 7 h/day, 5 days/week, for up to 18 months), Jones et al. (1994) also found that the mass of chrysotile in the lungs increased for several months and then appeared to decline, although exposure continued, in agreement with the Wagner et al. study (1974). Oberdörster (1994), using various types of published data, including a 30-month exposure of baboons (Oberdörster & Lehnert, 1991), calculated that the chrysotile clearance half-times in monkeys are in the order of 90–100 days.

Limited information exists concerning the effect of cigarette smoke on the lung clearance of asbestos fibre. Muhle et al. (1983) investigated the effect of cigarette smoke on the retention of UICC chrysotile A and UICC crocidolite in rats. Results showed a doubling of crocidolite fibres in the lungs of the groups exposed to cigarette smoke compared with animals not exposed to cigarette smoke. A plateau was found for chrysotile, as in the study of Wagner et al. (1974), but this was not influenced by cigarette smoke. This difference between the two fibre types can be explained by a higher deposition rate of chrysotile in the upper airways by interception compared with crocidolite and a decrease in deep lung clearance induced by cigarette smoke. Lippmann et al. (1980) showed that tracheobronchial clearance in humans is influenced by cigarette smoke and Cohen et al. (1979) and Bohning et al. (1982) showed that long-term smoking reduces long-term deep lung clearance.

Several studies have shown that short fibres are generally cleared at faster rates than long fibres. In their inhalation experiment, Kauffer et al. (1987) exposed rats to UICC Canadian chrysotile for 5 h at 5 mg/m^3. Animals were killed at different intervals over the subsequent 90 days and their lungs lavaged. In the lung tissue, the prevalence of fibres less than 5 µm in length decreased while that of fibres longer than 5 µm increased with post-exposure time. An opposite pattern of distribution was observed in the bronchoalveolar lavage (BAL) fluids. This indicates that fibres greater than 5 µm in length are cleared less efficiently from the rat lung than fibres less than 5 µm in length.

Davis (1989) also found that short fibres (< 10 µm in length) are cleared more rapidly than long fibres (> 10 µm in length). In his study, rats were exposed by inhalation to chrysotile or amosite fibres at 10 mg/m^3 for 12 months. The lung clearance percentages over a 6-month period after exposure were 55 and 90% for long and short chrysotile fibres, respectively. The lung clearance percentages for long and short amosite fibres were 14 and 20%, respectively.

In the study by Abraham et al. (1988), referred to previously in this section, the mean length of chrysotile fibres increased during the 90 days from 5 to 13 µm with a reduction in fibre diameter from 0.13 to 0.09 µm due to fibre splitting. Crocidolite fibres remained practically unchanged (mean length 6.2 to 5.7 µm and mean diameter 0.12 to 0.10 µm). These findings indicate that shorter chrysotile fibres will be preferentially cleared and that with time the proportion of thinner fibres increases due to fibre splitting.

The observation that chrysotile fibres undergo longitudinal splitting is supported by many other studies. In a study of the number and dimensions of chrysotile fibres in rat lungs following short inhalation exposures, Roggli & Brody (1984) found that the Mg:Si ratio of chrysotile fibres did not differ significantly from that of the original material. Over a period of 1 month there was a decline both in the numbers of fibres in lung and in the estimated total mass of chrysotile remaining. The mean length of the residual fibres appeared to increase. The mean fibre diameter decreased, which suggests that chrysotile fibres were splitting longitudinally into smaller groups of fibrils.

Coin et al. (1992, 1994) found that chrysotile fibres > 16 µm in length were not cleared at a significant rate from the rat lung over a 30-day period following a 3-h inhalation exposure. They found that the average diameter of retained fibres decreased over time, consistent with longitudinal splitting, and that the average length of retained fibres increased over time, consistent with slower clearance of longer fibres. The authors attributed the failure of these long fibres to be cleared from the lung to the inability of pulmonary macrophages to engulf them.

Le Bouffant et al. (1987) exposed rats to 5 mg/m^3 of chrysotile B for 24 months. They found that most of the fibres had undergone splitting by the end of the inhalation period and that chrysotile fibre numbers rapidly declined following inhalation.

Kimizuka et al. (1987), who administered chrysotile and amosite fibres by intratracheal instillation to hamsters, found initially a rapid reduction in the ratio of short to long chrysotile fibres, indicating faster clearance of short fibres. At 2 years, however, the proportion of short fibres had increased again to more than 50%. This is most likely due to breaking up of the longer and thicker fibres in the lungs. This notion was supported by the decrease in diameter of chrysotile with time. Amosite showed progressive reduction in the proportion of short fibres in the lung tissue, which was not reversed with time.

The numbers of chrysotile fibres remaining in the lung over a 2-year period, following their administration by intratracheal instillation, were measured by Bellmann et al. (1987). Virgin UICC chrysotile A was used, as well as the same material from which the magnesium had been removed by leaching with oxalic acid *in vitro*. As shown in Fig. 6,

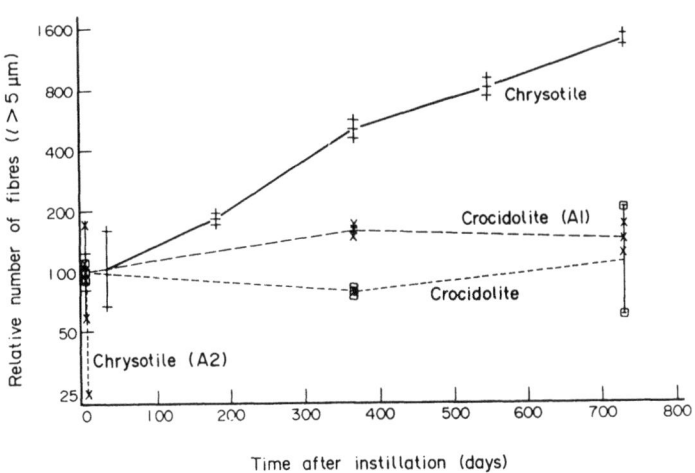

Fig. 6. Relative number of asbestos fibres longer than 5 μm in the lung ash at different sacrifice dates. A1: pretreatment with 0.1 M oxalic acid, 24 h, 20°C; A2: pretreatment with 0.1 M oxalic acid, 39 h, 60°C (Bellmann et al., 1987)

the number of intact chrysotile fibres longer than 5 µm increased by a factor of about 15 over the 2-year duration of the study. A significant reduction in the mean diameter of fibres > 5 µm in length was observed, which provides evidence of fibre splitting. The magnesium-leached fibres were removed from the rat lung with a half-time of only 2 days.

Coffin et al. (1992) administered large amounts of chrysotile fibres (6-32 mg) to the rat by intratracheal instillation and measured retention. There was an apparent increase in fibre numbers between 1 and 10 days after instillation, which the authors attributed to the splitting of fibre bundles. After this initial period there was no significant further change in the numbers of Stanton fibres (equal to or greater than 8 µm in length and equal to or less than 0.25 µm in diameter). However, the doses administered may well have been sufficient to overload macrophage-mediated clearance of fibres from the alveolar region of the lung.

5.1.4 Fibre translocation

Available experimental evidence indicates that chrysotile fibres can be transported through the epithelium with subsequent migration to the interstitium. Information on the movement of chrysotile fibres from the lung parenchyma to either the parietal or visceral pleura is conflicting. While chrysotile fibres have been detected in pleural tissues of workers who died of asbestos-related diseases in several studies, other studies did not show this. Additionally, chrysotile fibres were not found in the rat pleura in an acute inhalation study.

5.1.4.1 Fibre translocation in humans

In a study of asbestos fibres in the lung parenchyma and the parietal pleura of 29 asbestos workers, Sebastien et al. (1980) found that chrysotile fibres predominated in the pleura and that amphibole fibres could not be detected. A similar result was reported by Dodson et al. (1990). Kohyama & Suzuki (1991) found short chrysotile fibres in pleural plaques and in mesothelial tumours. In contrast, Boutin et al. (1993) found 0.21×10^6 fibres per g of parietal pleura and 1.96×10^6 in samples of lung parenchyma. Fibre concentrations were higher in subjects with a history of asbestos exposure and most of the fibres were amphiboles. Churg (1994) reported detection of chrysotile fibres in the subpleural parenchyma in chrysotile miners and millers. Kobayashi et al. (1987) reported the detection of few asbestos fibres as asbestos bodies in the extrathoracic organs (pancreas, spleen, etc.) of human subjects exposed to chrysotile.

5.1.4.2   *Fibre translocation in animal models*

In the inhalation study of Brody et al. (1981), the examination of tissues by electron microscopy revealed that chrysotile fibres deposited at the bifurcations of the alveolar ducts were taken up not only by alveolar macrophages but also by type I epithelial cells during the 1-h inhalation exposure. Some days after exposure, fibres were found in interstitial macrophages and fibroblasts. These observations suggest that there may be direct fibre penetration of the epithelial surface and that chrysotile fibrils can be transported to the interstitium through type I epithelial cells.

Oghiso et al. (1984) exposed rats by intermittent inhalation to chrysotile fibres (95% < 6 µm in length, no fibre > 0.5 µm diameter) or crocidolite fibres (98.7% < 5 µm in length, 4.2% > 0.5 µm diameter) for 3 months and then killed them after 2–16 months. Electron microscopy revealed some similarities, but also distinct differences in the pulmonary distribution of the two types of fibre. Thickened alveolar duct bifurcations, associated with aggregates of macrophages, were seen long after exposure ceased, but crocidolite-exposed rats also had subpleural collections of alveolar macrophages, many of which contained crocidolite fibres.

Coin et al. (1992) exposed rats to chrysotile fibres by inhalation for 3 h (see section 5.1.2) killing them at times up to 29 days following exposure. The authors found no evidence of translocation of chrysotile fibres to the pleura. They did find, however, substantial numbers of inhaled fibres deposited within 1–2 mm of the visceral pleura of the rat.

The fate of chrysotile (mean length 3.6 µm, mean diameter 0.05 µm), crocidolite (mean length 2.5 µm, mean diameter 0.14 µm) and glass fibres, following injection into the pleural cavity of rats, was studied by Bignon et al. (1979). By 90 days after injection, fibres were found at similar concentrations in lung, liver, kidney and brain, while in the thoracic lymph nodes the concentrations were higher. The authors concluded that the majority of fibres can migrate rapidly from the site of administration, principally via the pulmonary lymphatics. In the case of chrysotile, particularly, the mean length of fibres found in the lung parenchyma was greater than that of the administered material. In view of the way the fibres were administered in this study, the relevance of the results to prediction of the behaviour of fibres following inhalation may be limited.

5.1.5 Mechanisms of fibre clearance

There is considerable uncertainty about the mechanisms responsible for the more rapid removal of chrysotile fibres from the lung than in the case of amphibole asbestos fibres. It is uncertain whether the more effective removal of chrysotile fibres is due to more rapid fibre dissolution or to more rapid clearance of shorter fibres as a result of breakage. Another explanation may be movement and dispersion in the watery atmosphere in the lung.

Most of the evidence for the preferential dissolution of magnesium from chrysotile is derived from measurement of the magnesium/silicon ratio of fibres recovered from lung using analytical electron microscopy. A reduction in the Mg/Si ratio measured in fibres recovered from human lung was first reported by Langer et al. (1970). Subsequently, Jaurand et al. (1977) found that the extent of magnesium depletion varied from one fibre to another and even along the axis of the same fibre. Sebastien et al. (1986b) examined chrysotile fibres longer than 5 µm and thicker than 0.1 µm and found magnesium depletion as high as 50%. On the other hand, Churg & DePaoli (1988) found only slight magnesium depletion in fibres recovered from the lung of chrysotile miners many years after their last exposure.

One possible explanation for the diversity of results is the impossibility of measuring Mg:Si ratios at a resolution applicable to individual chrysotile fibrils. In relatively thick chrysotile fibres, only the fibrils near the surface of a bundle will be subjected to leaching and those in the interior may remain intact. Another factor is that, once leaching occurs, the unsupported silica structure on the outside of a fibril may disintegrate and this may impose an upper limit to estimates of magnesium depletion based on Mg:Si ratios (Morgan, 1994). Hume & Rimstidt (1992) have proposed that the brucite layer of chrysotile dissolves in the lung leaving the silica layer exposed; this then dissolves at a slower rate and it is suggested that this is the rate-controlling step. These authors developed a "shrinking-fibre model", which predicts that a chrysotile fibre 1 μm in diameter will dissolve completely in 9 ± 4.5 months.

Results of available experimental studies also gave conflicting evidence with regard to magnesium depletion. For example, Jones et al. (1994) obtained values for magnesium depletion ranging from 10 to 40%. Kimizuka et al. (1987) reported magnesium depletion in the lung of hamsters. On the other hand, Coin et al. (1994) found no significant leaching of magnesium over a period of 30 days following administration of chrysotile to rats by inhalation, and Churg et al. (1989) reported a similar result with guinea-pigs following intratracheal instillation.

Bellman et al. (1987) showed that magnesium is removed from chrysotile fibres following their administration to rats by intratracheal instillation and that leaching rates are much greater during the first month than subsequently. These authors also showed that chrysotile fibres, from which the magnesium had been removed by prior treatment with oxalic acid *in vitro,* were removed from the lung with a half-time of only a few days. This explains the observation that the carcinogenic potency of magnesium-leached chrysotile is much reduced, or eliminated completely, compared with that of the untreated fibre (Morgan et al., 1977; Monchaux et al., 1981).

Limited information is available in support of the fibre fragmentation hypothesis. Churg et al. (1993) showed that short chrysotile fibres are present in considerably larger numbers than long fibres in the lungs of chrysotile miners and millers even years after exposure has ceased. While this finding may reflect fragmentation of long inhaled fibres into shorter fibres, it might also reflect retention of some portion of the fibre burden in a sequestration compartment with no change in size distribution.

In summary, available data indicates that both fibre breakage and dissolution are likely mechanisms for the rapid removal of chrysotile fibres from the lung.

5.2 Ingestion

An important question in the evaluation of the possible risks associated with the ingestion of chrysotile asbestos is whether fibres can migrate from the lumen into and through the walls of the gastro-intestinal tract to be distributed within the body and subsequently cleared.

Review of the available data has been published in Environmental Health Criteria 53 (IPCS, 1986). The main conclusions were:

(a) It is not possible to conclude with certainty that chrysotile fibres do not cross the gastrointestinal wall. However, available evidence indicates that, if penetration does occur, it is extremely limited (Cook, 1983).

(b) There is no available information on bioaccumulation/retention of ingested chrysotile fibres. Simulated gastric juice has been shown to alter the physical and chemical properties of chrysotile fibres (Seshan, 1983).

(c) There was no difference in the level of urinary chrysotile between subjects drinking water with high compared to those drinking water with much lower natural chrysotile contamination (Boatman et al., 1983).

Finn & Hallenbeck (1985) investigated the number of chrysotile fibres in the urine of six workers occupationally exposed to chrysotile. The levels of chrysotile fibres in the urine of exposed workers were significantly higher than in a control group.

6. EFFECTS ON LABORATORY MAMMALS AND *IN VITRO* TEST SYSTEMS

6.1 Introduction

Several caveats are important in the interpretation of results of inhalation studies in laboratory animals and in cells *in vitro*. A search of the literature on the effects of chrysotile in experimental *in vivo* and *in vitro* models reveals few dose–response studies with appropriate positive and negative "control" dusts. Concentrations of chrysotile and other dusts used in inhalation experiments are several magnitudes higher than concentrations encountered in the workplace and environment today. Moreover, preparations of chrysotile and other dusts used in many experiments are poorly characterized. In the majority of studies before 1980, concentrations are expressed on a mass basis rather than on a fibre number basis. This may be misleading when comparing samples of chrysotile and amphibole asbestos, because the former may contain more than 10 times more fibres per unit weight.

There has been a great deal of debate concerning the relevance of various routes of exposure in experimental animals to risk assessment in humans (McClellan et al., 1992; IPCS, 1993). The general consensus is that all routes of administration should be considered, but that they should be given different weightings in relation to assessment of potential hazard to humans.

Positive results in an inhalation study on animals have important significance for the hazard evaluation of exposure to airborne fibres in humans. Strong arguments would need to be made against the relevance for humans of such a finding. However, the lack of a response in an inhalation study on animals does not mean that the material is not hazardous for humans. For instance, rats, being obligate nose-breathers, have a greater filtering capacity than humans.

As discussed by IPCS (1988), a negative result in a properly conducted intratracheal study would suggest that a given type of fibre may not be hazardous for parenchymal lung tissue. A positive result, however, would require further study since the normal filtering capacity of the respiratory tract has been bypassed. However, pulmonary clearance mechanisms are intact. The results of studies involving intrapleural injection or implantation and intraperitoneal injection should be viewed in a similar way to intratracheal instillation studies. With these methods, both filtering and clearance mechanisms are compromised. Such studies may be more sensitive than inhalation studies because a higher number of fibres can be introduced. Therefore, a negative result would be highly relevant, but a positive result should be confirmed by further investigation.

6.2 Effects on laboratory mammals

6.2.1 *Summary of previous studies*

The results of early inhalation experiments were presented in Environmental Health Criteria 53 (IPCS, 1986). Fibrosis has been observed in many species following inhalation of chrysotile. In several studies there was progression of fibrosis following cessation of exposure (Wagner et al., 1974, 1980; Wehner et al., 1979). In the majority of the studies only the airborne mass concentrations were measured; the numbers and size distributions were not considered. Shorter fibres were found to be less fibrogenic (Davis et al., 1980).

Unlike fibrosis, which has been observed in several animal species following inhalation of chrysotile, a consistently increased incidence of lung tumours or pleural mesothelioma has been observed only in the rat. Rats with lung tumours had significantly more fibrosis than those without (Wagner et al., 1974). In a study with exposure to approximately 10 mg/m^3 of three amphibole and two chrysotile asbestos types, Wagner et al. (1974) found 11 mesotheliomas, 4 of which occurred following exposure to Canadian but none following exposure to Rhodesian chrysotile. Davis et al. (1978) compared amosite, crocidolite and Rhodesian chrysotile at 10 mg/m^3 as well as at equal fibre numbers (fibres > 5 µm in length). Both by mass and by fibre number, chrysotile proved the most fibrogenic and carcinogenic, but the authors pointed out that, while numbers of fibres longer than 5 µm were roughly equal, the chrysotile dust cloud had many more very long fibres (> 20 µm in length).

Effects on Laboratory Mammals and In Vitro Test Systems

Since it became obvious that relatively few mesotheliomas developed in rats following asbestos inhalation and since Wagner (1962) had shown that they could be induced by direct dust injection into body cavities, the injection technique has been frequently used. The results of such early experiments were summarized by IPCS (1986). The major finding from these studies is that, following injection, short fibres are less fibrogenic (Burger & Engelbrecht, 1970; Davis, 1972) and that the most carcinogenic fibres are > 8 µm in length and < 0.25 µm in diameter (Stanton & Wrench, 1972; Pott & Friedrichs, 1972; Pott et al., 1972, 1976; Stanton et al., 1977). Short fibres show little carcinogenicity. The numbers of mesotheliomas produced in these studies were high (up to 90% of animals). Several authors reported a clear dose–response effect (Smith et al., 1968; Stanton & Wrench, 1972; Wagner et al., 1973).

The ability of asbestos to cause gastrointestinal cancer following ingestion has been examined in many experimental studies reviewed extensively by Condie (1983) and Toft et al. (1984). Early studies on ingested asbestos were reviewed by IPCS (1986). There was no conclusive evidence of either histopathological or biochemical effects on the gastrointestinal wall, or of carcinogenicity in the animal species studied.

6.2.2 Recent long-term inhalation studies

The results of the more recent inhalation studies in various animal species are presented in Table 18.

In an inhalation study on rats (10 mg/m^3 UICC chrysotile B for up to 12 months), Wagner et al. (1984) observed a mean fibrosis grade 4.1 and a 25% incidence of adenomas and carcinomas. Le Bouffant et al. (1987), using Canadian chrysotile as a positive control in experiments with MMM(V)Fs in rats (5 mg/m^3 chrysotile B, 5 h/day, 5 days/week for 24 months), reported unquantified fibrosis and pulmonary tumours in 21% of male and 17% of female rats. Muhle et al. (1987), exposing rats to 6 mg/m^3 Calidria chrysotile 5 h/day, four times each week for 12 months, reported the presence of pulmonary fibrosis in 42% of rats, but found no pulmonary tumours.

Table 18. Long-term inhalation studies

Species	Group size	Protocol[a]	Results[a]	Reference
Rat	24 male, 24 female	Exposure: 10 mg/m³ UICC chrys B for up to 12 months. Used as a positive control in experiments with MMM(V)F.	Mean fibrosis grade 4.1 (Wagner scale). Adenomas and carcinomas 12/48 (25%).	Wagner et al., 1984
Rat (Sprague-Dawley)	150 male	Exposure: 1.0 mg/m³ chrys 7 h/day, 5 days/week, for 18 months. Ball milled. Concentration of airborne fibres >5 µm in length was 0.79 f/cm³.	No fibrosis or tumours at 24 months.	Platek et al, 1985
Monkey	10	Exposure: 1.0 mg/m³ chrys 7 h/day, 5 days/week, for 18 months. Ball milled. Concentration of airborne fibres >5 µm in length was 0.79 f/cm³.	No fibrosis (estimated by biopsy) at 28 months.	Platek et al, 1985
Rat	24 male, 23 female	Exposure: 5 mg/m³ chrys B 5 h/day, 5 days/week for 24 months. Used as a positive control in experiments with MMM(V)F.	Fibrosis reported in chrys group but not quantified. Pulmonary tumours in 5/24 (21%) male rats and in 4/23 (17%) female rats.	Le Bouffant et al., 1987
Rat (Wistar)	48 male	Exposure: 10 mg/m³ tremolite or brucite 7 h/day, 5 days/week for 12 months.	Tremolite very fibrogenic. Pulmonary tumours and mesotheliomas in 20/39 (51%) rats. Brucite caused mild fibrosis. Pulmonary tumours in 5/38 (13%) rats.	Davis et al, 1985

Table 18 (contd).

Species	Number	Exposure	Results	Reference
Rat (Wistar)	48 male	Exposure: 7 h/day, 5 days/week for 12 months; mean conc. of WDC samples 5 mg/m³, concentration of chrys yarn 4.3 mg/m³.	All chrys samples very fibrogenic. Pulmonary tumours and mesotheliomas in 16/42 (38%) for standard chrys, 18/41 (44%), 18/37 (49%), 21/43 (49%), 21/44 (48%) for WDC preparations.	Davis et al., 1986a
Rat (Wistar)	48 male	Exposure: 10 mg/m³ of respirable dust 7 h/day, 5 days/week for 12 months. Long fibre amos: cloud generated from raw material. Short fibre amos: very few fibres > 5 µm in length.	Long amos extremely fibrogenic. Pulmonary tumours and mesotheliomas in 13/40 (33%). Short amos no fibrosis. No pulmonary tumours or mesotheliomas.	Davis et al., 1986b
Rat (Wistar)	50 female	Exposure: 6 mg/m³ of Calidria chrys 5 h/day, 4 times each week for 12 months. Used as a positive control in experiments with MMM(V)F.	Some septal fibrosis in 21/50 (42%) rats. No pulmonary tumours.	Muhle et al., 1987
Rat (Wistar)	48 male	Exposure: 10 mg/m³ 7 h/day, 5 days/week for 12 months. Long fibre chrys: cloud generated from raw chrys. Short fibre chrys: fibres >5 µm reduced 5 times; fibres >30 µm reduced 80 times.	Long fibre chrys very fibrogenic. Pulmonary tumours and mesotheliomas in 23/40 (58%) rats.	Davis & Jones, 1988

Table 18 (contd).

Species	Group size	Protocol[a]	Results[a]	Reference
Rat (Wistar)	48 male	Exposure: 10 mg/m^3 7 h/day, 5 days/week for 12 months. Two clouds of UICC chrys A, one of which had reduced electrostatic charge by exposure to ionizing radiation from a thallium-204 source of beta particles.	Interstitial fibrosis reduced by 38% in "discharged" group compared to standard chrys. Pulmonary tumours and mesotheliomas in 11/39 (28%) rats in "discharged" group; 14/36 (11%) rats in standard chrys group.	Davis et al., 1988
Rat (Wistar)	48 male	Exposure: 10 mg/m^3 7 h/day, 5 days/week for 12 months. Six treatment groups, UICC chrys A or UICC amosite alone or mixed with either 10 mg/m^3 of titanium dioxide or 2 mg/m^3 of quartz.	Advanced fibrosis increased for both asbestos types by addition of quartz but not by titanium dioxide. Pulmonary tumours and mesotheliomas: chrys 13/37 (35%) rats, chrys + TiO$_2$ 26/41 (51%) rats, chrys + quartz 22/38 (58%) rats; amos 14/40 (35%) rats, amos + TiO$_2$ 20/40 (50%) rats, amos + quartz 26/39 (67%) rats.	Davis et al., 1991a
Rat (Fisher 344)	63	Exposure: 10 mg/m^3 chrys A 6 h/day, 5 days/week for 24 months. Used as a positive control in experiments with MMM(V)F.	Mean fibrosis grade 4.0 (Wagner scale). Pulmonary tumours and mesotheliomas 13/63 (21%) rats.	Bunn et al., 1993
Hamster	100 male	Exposure: 11 mg/m^3 chrys B 6 h/day, 5 days/week for 18 months. Used as a positive control in experiments with MMM(V)F.	Mean fibrosis grade 4.3 (Wagner scale) at 3 months. No pulmonary tumours or mesotheliomas.	Hesterberg et al., 1991

Table 18 (contd).

Baboon		Exposure: 6 h/day, 5 days/week for up to 4 years		Goldstein & Coetzee, 1990
	21	1) UICC chrysotile A, exposure not specified	1) No mesotheliomas	
	18	2) UICC amosite 1100 f/cm^3, exposure for 4 years	2) 1/18 (5.6%) animals with mesothelioma	
	78	3) UICC crocidolite 1130-14 000 f/cm^3, exposure for 1.5-3 years	3) 3/78 (3.8%) animals with mesothelioma	
Baboon		Exposure: 6 h/day, 5 days/week		Hiroshima et al., 1993
	4	1) UICC chrysotile A 106,074-368,772 f/cm^3 for 8.5-24 months	1) No mesothelioma	
	5	2) UICC amosite 997,678 f/cm^3 for 49 months (dose that produced mesothelioma)	2) 2/5 animals with mesothelioma	
	5	3) crocidolite (Transvaal or UICC) 432,291 f/cm^3 for 15 months 769,784 f/cm^3 for 35 months (dose that produced mesothelioma)	3) 2/5 animals with mesothelioma	

[a] chrys = chrysotile; MMM(V)F = man-made mineral (vitreous) fibres; WDC = wet dispersed chrysotile; amos = amosite.

Davis et al. (1985) examined the effects on rats of tremolite and brucite, two materials frequently found as contaminants of commercially produced chrysotile (10 mg/m^3, 7 h/day, 5 days/week, for 12 months). A sample of asbestiform tremolite from Korea was highly fibrogenic and carcinogenic, while brucite was less hazardous. However, it was demonstrated that the sample which was supposedly brucite was contaminated with chrysotile fibres, and it was not possible to determine the relative pathogenicity of these two minerals.

The same group (Davis et al., 1986a) examined the long-term effects of dust from samples of wet dispersed chrysotile (WDC) in rats. WDC is a preparation used to produce textile yarn. Raw chrysotile is first separated into individual fibrils by treatment with detergents and then rebound with electrolytes while the slurry is extruded from a narrow nozzle. Handling this material liberates much less dust than standard chrysotile textile yarn. In the experimental studies, however, where respirable dust was produced by milling, both specimens of WDC dust and the parent chrysotile material (5 mg/m^3, 7 h/day, 5 days/week for 12 months) produced widespread fibrosis and pulmonary tumours in up to 50% of animals. One experimental WDC sample with relatively thick fibres produced as much disease at a dose level of only approximately 100 fibres/ml (> 5 μm in length, measured by PCOM) as was found in the other groups treated with WDC or standard chrysotile where dose levels were 500-650 fibres/ml. The authors concluded that WDC separates into fibrils in lung tissue more rapidly than standard chrysotile. The relatively few thick WDC fibres could generate as many long thin subunits as clouds of similar mass that originally contained more thin fibres.

Platek et al. (1985) treated rats and monkeys with a specially prepared short fibre sample of chrysotile for 18 months (the mass dose level was only 1 mg/m^3, of which < 1 fibre/ml was longer than 5 μm as measured by PCOM). After a total follow-up of 24 months the rats had developed neither fibrosis nor pulmonary tumours. No fibrosis was found in monkeys by open lung biopsies after 24 months. Davis et al. (1986b), exposing rats to amosite asbestos fibres (all fibres were < 5 μm in length), found no pulmonary carcinomas, while numbers of benign tumours and levels of pulmonary fibrosis were similar to those in control animals. In contrast, a dust cloud generated from raw amosite with many very long fibres was extremely fibrogenic and carcinogenic. Similar studies examined the importance of fibre length with inhaled Canadian chrysotile (Davis & Jones, 1988). Unfortunately, in this case, the "short" fibre chrysotile preparation did have a small proportion of long fibres, and fibrosis and pulmonary tumours did develop. However, a comparison cloud generated from the same original chrysotile sample, to maximize the number of long fibres, produced 5 times more fibrosis and 3 times more tumours for the same mass dose.

Airborne chrysotile asbestos is able to hold a high electrostatic charge, and there have been reports that this may effect fibre deposition in the lower pulmonary tract (Vincent et al., 1981; Jones et al., 1983). Consequently, Davis et al. (1988) treated rats with equal clouds of UICC Rhodesian chrysotile, either carrying the normal electrostatic charge or discharged by exposure to ionizing radiation from a thallium-204 source. Rats treated with discharged chrysotile had less fibrosis, tumours and retained chrysotile in their lung tissue, but not all these differences were statistically significant.

Davis et al. (1991a) examined the effect on rats of inhaling chrysotile or amosite asbestos (10 mg/m^3, 7 h/day, 5 days/week for 12 months) simultaneously with either titanium dioxide (10 mg/m^3) or quartz (2 mg/m^3). Increased levels of pulmonary fibrosis above levels produced by chrysotile or amosite alone were observed in combination with quartz, but not with addition of titanium dioxide. Tumour production was also increased, but in this case a combination of asbestos and titanium dioxide was as carcinogenic as a combination of asbestos and quartz. Of particular interest in this study was the finding of granulomas on the visceral pleural surface that contained both particles and asbestos fibres in animals treated with asbestos and quartz. Similar granulomas have not been reported in previous experiments with pure asbestos where fibres accumulated beneath the external elastic lamina of the lung and seldom penetrated to the pleural surface. The increased pleural penetration of asbestos fibres in coexposures with quartz dust was associated with increased production of mesotheliomas. The recorded proportions of mesotheliomas were higher than those previously reported in any experiments with commercial varieties of asbestos. Evidence of interspecies differences in response to asbestos and other mineral fibres has been reported. Hamsters treated with respirable refractory ceramic fibre developed no pulmonary carcinomas but 43% developed mesotheliomas. Chrysotile produced neither type of tumour in this species. The mass dose levels were 29 mg/m^3 for ceramic fibres and 11 mg/m^3 for chrysotile (6 h/day, 5 days/week for 18 months) (Hesterberg et al., 1991). Twenty-one percent of rats treated with Canadian chrysotile (10 mg/m^3, 6 h/day, 5 days/week for 24 months) developed both lung tumours (19% of animals) and mesothelioma (one rat)(Bunn et al., 1993; Hesterberg et al., 1993).

Studies in baboons suggest that chrysotile is less apt to cause mesothelioma in comparison to crocidolite and amosite asbestos. In two reports (Goldstein & Coetzee, 1990; Hiroshima et al., 1993), no mesotheliomas nor lung carcinomas were reported after exposure to chrysotile, although mesotheliomas were observed in amosite- and crocidolite-exposed baboons. However, the chrysotile exposure levels were lower than those of amosite or crocidolite in the latter study, while the level of chrysotile in the former study was not specified. Studies in baboons indicate that fibrosis is observed with UICC samples of chrysotile, amosite and crocidolite asbestos (Hiroshima et al., 1993). In all cases, the severity of fibrosis was directly related to cumulative dose.

In experimental inhalation studies with different fibre types it has been an almost universal finding that fibres that are very fibrogenic are also carcinogenic. Davis & Cowie (1990) emphasized this by reporting on advanced fibrosis in 144 rats, aged 2.5 years or more, that had been exposed to a number of different asbestos types, including Rhodesian and Canadian chrysotile. The 85 animals that had pulmonary tumours showed almost twice the level of advanced pulmonary fibrosis as the 59 animals that had not developed tumours.

6.2.3 *Intratracheal and intrabronchial injection studies*

Table 19 shows the results of intratracheal injection studies with chrysotile documenting fibrosis in sheep, rats and mice.

Table 19. Intratracheal injection studies (fibrogenicity)

Species	Dose and group size	Protocol	Results	Reference
Rats (Wistar, male)	UICC chrysotile B, short chrysotile (4T30) (1, 5, 10 mg) N = 5/group	Single exposure. Histopathology at 1-60 days and 8 months	Severe peribronchiolar fibrosis at all conc. with chrysotile B. No fibrosis with short chrysotile.	Lemaire, 1985, 1991; Lemaire et al., 1985, 1989
Mouse (Balb/c, sex not specified)	UICC chrysotile A (0.5 mg) number not specified	Single exposure. Histopathology at 0.5, 1, 2, 3, 6 and 9 months.	No severe fibrosis until 9 months.	Bissonnette et al., 1989
Sheep (male)	UICC Canadian chrysotile B (1, 10, 50, 100 mg) N = 6/group	Single exposure. Histopathology at 60 days	Fibrosis only in 100 mg group.	Begin et al., 1987
Sheep (male)	UICC chrysotile A, UICC crocidolite, latex beads (100 mg) N = 15/group	Single exposure. Histopathology at 8 months.	Histological score for fibrosis = 1.9 ± 0.3 in crocidolite and 2.8 ± 1 in chrysotile groups.	Sebastien et al., 1990

At high doses (100 mg) of chrysotile administered via intratracheal instillation in sheep, fibrosis appeared to be more marked with chrysotile than with crocidolite (Sebastien et al., 1990). However, the development of fibrosis exhibited evidence of an apparent threshold in this model, as fibrosis was not observed in sheep after injection of 1, 10 or 50 mg of chrysotile (Begin et al., 1987). Repeated instillations of 100 mg chrysotile over a 2-year period in sheep resulted in progression of fibrosis and lung infections (Begin et al., 1991).

Use of an intratracheal injection model in rats has yielded additional data suggesting the decreased fibrogenicity of short-fibre chrysotile (Lemaire, 1985, 1991; Lemaire et al., 1985, 1989). No fibrogenicity was observed with injections of short chrysotile at 1, 5 and 10 mg; however, UICC chrysotile B caused peribronchiolar fibrosis at all concentrations.

Intratracheal studies in mice indicated focal collagen deposition in mice exposed to chrysotile, but more severe fibrosis after exposure to quartz (Bissonnette et al., 1989). Collagen and elastin deposition per unit lung weight was greater after instillation of UICC chrysotile in comparison to UICC crocidolite (injected rats kept for a 12-month period after a single 1.6 mg injection) (Hirano et al., 1988).

The rat and sheep intratracheal injection models of fibrosis have also been used to elucidate the time frame of appearance of bombesin and vasoactive intestinal peptide (Day et al., 1985, 1987), populations of cells in bronchoalveolar lavage (BAL) (Lemaire, 1985), pulmonary function and alveolitis (Begin et al., 1985, 1986), and cytokines or inflammatory mediators (Lemaire et al., 1986a; Keith et al., 1987) in relationship to the development of fibrotic disease. The rat intratracheal injection model has also been used to assess the inflammatory and fibrogenic potential of other fibre types (xonotlite, Fibrefrax, attapulgite) in comparison to UICC chrysotile B and short chrysotile 4T30 (Lemaire et al., 1989). Overall, the order of reactivity was xonotlite < attapulgite < short chrysotile 4T30 < Fibrefrax < UICC chrysotile B.

Effects on Laboratory Mammals and In Vitro Test Systems

Intratracheal and intrabronchial injection studies on carcinogenicity are presented in Table 20. Studies by Coffin et al. (1992) evaluated UICC chrysotile A in comparison to UICC crocidolite and erionite. Large differences in the incidence of mesothelioma in intratracheal injection studies were demonstrated on the basis of tumour-to-fibre ratios based on lung burdens of fibres averaged from 1 day to 1 year. Erionite was 500-800 times more tumorigenic and crocidolite 30-60 times more tumorigenic than chrysotile on fibre number basis.

Other studies have examined the co-carcinogenic effects on rats of chrysotile in combination with benzo(a)pyrene (BP) (Fasske, 1988) or the systemic carcinogen N-nitrosoheptamethyleneimine (NHMI) and cadmium (Harrison & Heath, 1988). In the former study, BP appeared to be a weaker lung carcinogen than chrysotile. Synergistic effects of BP and chrysotile were not observed in comparison to chrysotile alone. In the latter study, the lung tumorigenic effects of chrysotile and NHMI appeared to be more than additive in comparison to those observed with NHMI or chrysotile alone.

Kimizuka et al. (1993) explored the co-carcinogenicity of chrysotile and amosite asbestos with BP in hamster lungs. Although tumours were not observed with either type of asbestos or BP alone, lung carcinomas occurred with chrysotile and BP (83%) and with amosite and BP (67%). The incidence of lung carcinomas in rats was higher when chrysotile was instilled repeatedly with the carcinogen N-bis(hydroxypropyl)nitrosamine (DHPN) (23/38 rats) than it was with chrysotile alone (1/31 rats) or chrysotile in combination with smoking (4/29 rats) (Yoshimura & Takemoto, 1991). Mesotheliomas were not observed with asbestos, smoking or DHPN alone, but were found in combination groups.

6.2.4 Intraperitoneal and intrapleural injection studies

The results of the most significant intraperitoneal and intrapleural injection studies are presented in Table 21.

Table 20. Intratracheal/intrabronchial injection studies (carcinogenicity)

Species	Dose and group size[a]	Protocol[a]	Results[a]	Reference
Rat (Fischer 344, male)	UICC chrys A (6, 16, 32 mg)[b]; N = 132 for 6 and 16 mg, 41 for 32 mg	21 weekly intratracheal instillations. Animals kept for lifespan.	At 6, 16 and 32 mg, % mesothelioma were 8.3, 7.5 and 9.8, % carcinoma were 27.3, 14.3 and 2.4, respectively No dose–response relationship.	Coffin et al., 1992
Rat (Wistar, both sexes)	1) Milled UICC chrys B (1 mg) 2) Benzo(a)pyrene (0.5 mg) 3) Chrys (1 mg) + BP (0.5 mg) N = 70-80/group	Single intrabronchial dose. Rats kept for 33 months.	1) 17/70 (24%) lung carcinomas and 1/70 (1.4%) mesothelioma 2) 7/78 (9%) lung carcinomas and 3/78 (4%) mesothelioma 3) 15/78 (19%) lung carcinomas and 1 mesothelioma.	Fasske, 1988
Rat (Lister hooded)	1) UICC chrys B (2 mg) 2) Chrys (2 mg) + cadmium (0.18 mg) 3) Chrys (2 mg) + NHMI (1 mg x10, s.c.) 4) Chrys (2 mg) + NHMI (1 mg x10, s.c.) + cadmium (0.18 mg) 5) NHMI (1 mg x10, s.c.)	Single intratracheal instillation of particular materials. 10 weekly subcutaneous administrations of NHMI	Lung tumours incidence: 1) Chrys alone 1/86 (1.2%) 2) NHMI alone 2/48 (4.2%) 3) Chrys + cadmium 1/94 (1.1%) 4) Chrys + NHMI 8/50 (16.6%) 5) Chrys + NHMI + cadmium 6/44 (13.6%)	Harrison & Heath, 1988

Table 20 (contd).

Species	Dose and group size[a]	Protocol[a]	Results[a]	Reference
Rat (Wistar)	1) Chrys (15 mg), N=31 2) DHPN (1 mg/kg bw) intraperitoneally, N=37 3) DHPN + chrys, N=38 4) chrys + smoke of 10 cigarettes, N=29 5) chrys + DHPN + smoke of 10 cigarettes, N=29	Single intratracheal dose of chrys, DHPN 3 intraperitoneal doses, exposure to smoke of 10 cigarettes/day, 6 days/week throughout lifespan.	Lung carcinomas: 1) 1/31 (3.2%) 2) 8/37 (21.6%) 3) 23/38 (60.5%) 4) 4/29 (13.8%) 5) 15/29 (51.7%) Mesotheliomas: 1) 0 2) 0 3) 8/38 (21.1%) 4) 2/29 (6.9%) 5) 4/29 (13.8%)	Yoshimura & Takemoto, 1991
Hamster	12/group 1) UICC chrys (0.2 mg) 2) UICC amos (0.2 mg) 3) BP (0.4 mg) 4) Chrys + BP 5) Amos + BP	Weekly intratracheal application through 6 weeks. Tumours examined 18 and 24 months after last instillation.	chrys, amos and BP alone: no tumours. 4) 16 carcinomas in 12 (83% of animals) 5) 11 carcinomas in 12 (68% of animals)	Kimizuka et al., 1993

[a] NHMI = N-nitrosoheptamethyleneimine, a relative systemic carcinogen; BP = benzo(a)pyrene; chrys = chrysotile; amos = amosite; DHPN = N-bis(2-hydroxypropyl) nitrosamine.
[b] Accumulated instilled doses. Equivalent to 6.5, 17.4 and 34.8 million fibres, respectively.

Table 21. Intrapleural and intraperitoneal injection studies

Species	Group size	Protocol[a]	Results[a,b]		Reference
Rat (Wistar, 20 males, 20 females)	40	Single intrapleural injection of 20 mg chrys, 1% >5 μm in length	Mesotheliomas in 14/32 (44%) rats (sexes unspecified)		Le Bouffant et al., 1985
Rat (Wistar, males)	24	Single intraperitoneal injection of 25 mg of 4 samples of WDC, 1 sample standard chrys	Mesotheliomas reported in 90% of rats in all groups (actual numbers unspecified). Median survival for WDC rats was 310-340 days, for standard chrys rats was 400 days		Davis et al., 1986a
Rat (Wistar, females)	32	Single intraperitoneal injection of:	Mesotheliomas	Median survival	Muhle et al., 1987
		Calidrian chrys (0.5 mg)	2/32 (6%)	812	
		Canadian chrys (1.0 mg)	27/32 (84%)	357	
Rat (Wistar, male)	24	Single intraperitoneal injection of:	Mesotheliomas	Median survival	Davis et al., 1986b
		long amosite (20 mg)	20/21	520	
		long amosite (10 mg)	21/24	535	
		short amosite (25 mg)	1/24	837	
		short amosite (10 mg)	0/24		
Rat (Wistar, male)	24	Single intraperitoneal injection of Canadian chrysotile:	Mesothelioma	Mean induction period	Davis & Jones, 1988
		long fibre (25 mg)	23/24 (96%)	361	
		long fibre (2.5 mg)	22/24 (92%)	511	
		long fibre (0.25 mg)	16/24 (67%)	736	

Table 21 (contd).

			Mesothelioma	Mean survival	
Rat (Wistar, female)		short fibre (25 mg)	22/24 (92%)	504	Pott et al., 1987
		short fibre (2.5 mg)	8/24 (33%)	675	
		short fibre (0.25 mg)	0/24 (0%)		
		Single intraperitoneal injection of:			
	34	UICC Rhodesian chrys (6 mg)	26/34 (76%)	497	
	34	UICC Rhodesian chrys (25 mg)	27/34 (79%)	420	
	34	UICC Rhodesian chrys (6 mg) (HCl treated)	0/34 (0%)		
	34	UICC Rhodesian chrys (25 mg) (HCl treated)	0/34 (0%)		
	39	UICC Rhodesian chrys milled (10 mg)	1/39 (2.6%)		
	32	UICC Canadian chrys (1.0 mg)	26/32 (81%)	392	
	30	UICC Canadian chrys (1.0 mg) + separate injection of PVNO	24/30 (80%)	462	
	32	Calidrian chrys (0.5 mg)	2/32 (6%)	742	
	36	UICC Canadian chrys (0.05 mg)	7/36 (19%)	448	
	34	UICC Canadian chrys (0.25 mg)	21/34 (62%)	406	
	36	UICC Canadian chrys (1.0 mg)	31/36 (86%)	245	

Table 21 (contd).

Species	Group size	Protocol[a]	Results[a,b]		Reference
Rat (Wistar, female)		Single intraperitoneal injection of:	Mesothelioma	(survival times not recorded)	Tilkes & Beck, 1989
	50	UICC Rhodesian chrys (2.0 mg)	25/50 (50%)		
	25	UICC Rhodesian chrys (10.0 mg)	14/25 (54%)		
	50	long asbestos-cement chrys (2.0 mg)	19/50 (38%)		
	25	long asbestos-cement chrys (10.0 mg)	8/25 (32%)		
	50	short asbestos-cement chrys (2.0 mg)	20/50 (40%)		
	25	short asbestos-cement chrys (10.0 mg)	8/25 (32%)		
	50	core asbestos-cement chrys (2.0 mg)	11/50 (22%)		
	25	core asbestos-cement chrys (10.0mg)	12/25 (48%)		
Rat (Wistar)					Yang et al., 1990
			Mesothelioma	Mean survival	
	53	Chinese chrys short (50 mg)	26/53 (49.1%)	630	
	52	Chinese chrys long (50 mg)	38/52 (73.1%)	647	
	51	Chinese croc short (50 mg)	23/51 (45.1%)	636	
	54	Chinese croc long (50 mg)	40/54 (74.1%)	492	

Table 21 (contd).

	3	UICC chrys (50 mg)	7/13 (53.8%)	550	
	13	UICC croc (50 mg)	8/13 (61.5%)	586	
	14	UICC glass fibre (50 mg)	10/14 (71.4%)	605	
	32	Saline control (2 x 1 ml)	0/32	726	
Rat (Wistar, male)		Single intraperitoneal injection of UICC Rhodesian chrysotile:	Mesothelioma	Median survival	Davis et al., 1991b
	24	15.0 mg	19/24 (79%)	476	
	24	10.0 mg	20/24 (83%)	476	
	24	7.5 mg	20/24 (83%)	516	
	24	5.0 mg	19/24 (79%)	506	
	32	2.5 mg	22/32 (69%)	613	
	32	0.5 mg	26/32 (81%)	693	
	32	0.05 mg	12/32 (38%)	903	
	48	0.01 mg	2/48 (4%)	NA	
Rat (Wistar, male)	33 or 36	Single intraperitoneal injection of tremolite:	Mesothelioma	Median survival	Davis et al., 1991c
		Californian (asbestiform)	36/36 (100%)	301	
		Swansea (asbestiform)	35/36 (97%)	365	
		Korea (asbestiform)	32/33 (97%)	428	
		Italy (non-asbestiform)	24/36 (67%)	755	
		Carr Brae (non-asbestiform)	4/33 (12%)	NA	
		Shinness (non-asbestiform)	2/36 (6%)	NA	

Table 21 (contd).

Species	Group size	Protocol[a]	Results[a,b]		Reference
Rat (Sprague-Dawley, male)	40	Single intrapleural injection of: Standard Canadian chrys (20 mg)	Mesothelioma 11/40 (28%)	Mean survival 632	Van der Meeren et al., 1992
		Phosphorylated Canadian chrys (20 mg) (3 samples)	11/40 (28%) 13/40 (33%) 16/40 (40%)	Median survival 612 to 642	
Rat (Fischer 344, male)	50/dose	Single intrapleural injection of: UICC Rhodesian chrys UICC croc UICC erionite [NB. Number of chrys fibres (length > 8 µm, diameter < 0.25 µm) was over 100 times higher than for croc or erionite]	Mesothelioma 118/142 (83%) 65/142 (45%) 137/144 (95%)		Coffin et al., 1992

[a] chrys = chrysotile; PVNO = polyvinyl-pyridine-N-oxide; asb = asbestos; croc = crocidolite; NA = not assessed.
[b] All survival or induction periods are given in days.

When Davis et al. (1986a) treated rats by intraperitoneal injection of a series of four wet dispersed chrysotile (WDC) preparations (see section 6.2.2) and a standard chrysotile sample, mesotheliomas were induced in over 90% of animals. The mean induction period of WDC preparations was 310-340 days, shorter than that for standard chrysotile. It was suggested by the authors that this was due to the rapid separation of WDC fibre bundles in the tissue. Muhle et al. (1987) included two samples of chrysotile in intraperitoneal tests along with man-made fibres. While Canadian chrysotile produced mesotheliomas in 84% of animals (dose of 1.0 mg), a sample of chrysotile from Calidria produced only 6% mesotheliomas (dose of 0.5 mg). Calidrian chrysotile consists of thick and often agglomerated bundles which are difficult to separate and size. Tilkes & Beck (1989) examined the carcinogenicity of chrysotile fibres separated from asbestos-cement sheeting by single intraperitoneal injection in rats. At doses of 2.0 and 10.0 mg both weathered and unweathered chrysotile materials produced similar number of mesotheliomas to raw chrysotile. The incidences of mesothelioma were not dose-related.

Le Bouffant et al. (1985) examined the carcinogenicity of "short" chrysotile fibres by intrapleural injection of 20 mg in 40 rats. Mesotheliomas were induced in 44% of animals, but the dust sample contained over 1% of fibres > 5 µm in length. Davis & Jones (1988) administered to six groups of 24 rats by a single intraperitoneal injection "long" and "short" chrysotile samples at doses of 0.25, 2.5 and 25 mg. All animals were followed practically throughout their life span. At 25 mg, samples of long and short chrysotile produced similar numbers of mesotheliomas (> 90%). At 2.5 mg, the long chrysotile material produced almost the same proportion of mesotheliomas while the short material produced tumours in only 33% of animals. At 0.25 mg, the long chrysotile still produced 67% of mesotheliomas while the short chrysotile produced none. The mean mesothelioma induction period was dose-dependent and significantly longer with short fibre preparations. In fact, it is difficult to conclude whether the zero mesothelioma incidence with short fibre exposure at the dose of 0.25 mg was an exposure threshold or the consequence of an induction period longer than the follow-up period. While in this study samples of long and short chrysotile fibres produced similar number of mesotheliomas at the dose of 25 mg, the same group of authors (Davis et al., 1986b) had previously reported that the intraperitoneal injection of 25 mg of amosite with all fibres shorter than 5 μm produced only a single mesothelioma in 24 rats. The authors attributed this difference to the presence of a small but significant number of long fibres in the "short" chrysotile sample.

Pott et al. (1987) examined the carcinogenicity of many mineral samples, including several chrysotile preparations, in a large intraperitoneal injection study on rats. It was reported that UICC Canadian chrysotile exhibited a clear dose–response effect over a dose range of 0.05 to 1.0 mg, although Rhodesian chrysotile showed no difference between doses of 6 and 25 mg. Milled UICC Rhodesian chrysotile produced only 2.6% mesotheliomas at a dose level of 10 mg, and treatment with hydrochloric acid eliminated the carcinogenic potential of Rhodesian chrysotile completely. Injecting the animals with polyvinyl-pyridine-N-oxide (PVNO) after an injection of UICC Canadian chrysotile had no effect on carcinogenicity. The results were confirmed in a further study by the same group of authors (Pott et al., 1989). These authors emphasized that the maximum carcinogenic potency of fibres is reached at a fibre length of ≥ 20 μm.

Davis et al. (1991b) reported detailed dose–response studies following intraperitoneal injection of UICC Rhodesian chrysotile, UICC crocidolite, UICC amosite and erionite in rats. Dose levels ranged from 0.005 to 25 mg, and a clear dose–response effect was seen for all four minerals. Only two mesotheliomas were recorded with the lowest chrysotile dose (0.01 mg), which contained 55.8×10^6 fibres of all lengths and 872 000 fibres > 8 μm in length. When the dose–response was considered by mass, erionite and chrysotile appeared significantly more carcinogenic than amosite or crocidolite. When considered by fibre number (fibres > 8 μm in length), chrysotile, amosite and crocidolite appeared similar, but erionite showed significantly higher carcinogenicity. In this study, fibres were sized by SEM.

In a similar comparison of fibre number and carcinogenicity by intrapleural injection, Coffin et al. (1992) counted and sized fibres by TEM. A dose level of 20 mg chrysotile produced similar numbers of mesotheliomas in rats (83%) to erionite and twice the proportion of mesotheliomas produced by crocidolite (45%). However, the chrysotile fibre numbers (> 8 µm in length) were reported to be 100 times greater than in the crocidolite preparation and 500 times greater than in erionite.

Van der Meeren et al. (1992) treated rats by intrapleural injection of either standard chrysotile or three samples of phosphorylated chrysotile at the same dose. There were no significant differences in mesothelioma production but the unphosphorylated chrysotile was reported to have at most half the number of "Stanton" size fibres per mg compared to the phosphorylated materials.

Pott (1994) evaluated results from carcinogenicity studies in rats and lung cancer risk data in humans. He concluded that there is no evidence of a lower carcinogenic potency of chrysotile fibre compared to amphibole asbestos fibres.

Because tremolite contamination of chrysotile is believed by some to enhance its pathogenicity, an injection study by Davis et al. (1991c) is of interest. Six tremolite samples (three of asbestiform type and three non-asbestiform varieties) were administered to rats by intraperitoneal injection. The three asbestiform preparations produced mesotheliomas in over 90% of animals, while the non-asbestiform samples produced a lower response which appeared to be related to the number of elongated spicules in the dust. Two preparations, with relatively few of these spicules, produced only a few mesotheliomas similar in numbers to those found in control rats.

6.2.5 Ingestion studies

The main chrysotile-related findings, reported in the Environmental Health Criteria 53 (IPCS, 1986), are as follows:

(a) There were no consistent pathological findings in the gastrointestinal tract of rats that had consumed up to 250 mg chrysotile per week for periods up to 25 months (Bolton et al., 1982), although some evidence of cellular damage was observed in the intestinal mucosa of rats fed 50 mg of chrysotile per day (Jacobs et al., 1978).

(b) In six identified studies on rats with chrysotile fed in diet (250 mg per week for up to 25 months, or 10% in diet over lifetime, or 1% short-range or 1% intermediate-range chrysotile fed to nursing mothers and over the lifetime of pups) (Donham et al.,1980; Bolton et al.,1982; McConnell, 1982; NTP, 1985), there was no significant treatment-related increase of carcinoma incidence. Only benign tumours of the large intestine were found in rats, fed with an intermediate range of chrysotile fibres, in the NTP study. Of special significance is the finding that no increase in tumour incidence was observed following administration of short-range chrysotile fibres, composed of size ranges similar to those found in drinking-water (McConnell, 1982; NTP, 1985).

Since the publication of Environmental Health Criteria 53 (IPCS, 1986), there have been only a few studies in which possible harmful effects of the ingestion of chrysotile asbestos have been examined in experimental animals. All these studies gave negative findings. McConnell et al. (1983) treated over 3000 hamsters (equal numbers of males and females) with various preparations of chrysotile and amosite in special food pellets containing 1% by weight of asbestos. Neither the male nor the female asbestos-treated groups showed a statistically significant increase in neoplasia in any tissue or organ compared to control groups. A study on Swiss albino male mice, fed orally with chrysotile asbestos suspended in water at a dosage of 20 mg/kg per day during 60 days, did not show induction of chromosomal aberrations or sperm abnormalities (Rita & Reddi, 1986). The most recent completed experimental ingestion study was reported by Truhaut & Chouroulinkov (1989). These authors fed groups of 70 rats with either chrysotile or a mixture of chrysotile and crocidolite (75:25) in palm oil at dose levels of 10, 60 or 360 mg per day for 2 years. No increase in tumour incidence in the treated animals was found compared to controls. Aberrant crypt foci were induced in rats given chrysotile by gavage at a dosage of 70 mg/kg per day (Corpet et al., 1993).

The subject of asbestos ingestion has been reviewed by Davis (1993), Polissar (1993) and Valić & Beritić-Stahuljak (1993).

6.3 Studies on cells

Cell cultures and cells from bronchioalveolar lavage (BAL) of animals or humans exposed to asbestos have been used to document the cytotoxicity and genotoxicity of asbestos preparations as well as other effects on cells, i.e. proliferative alterations, production of cytokines, which may be predictive of disease. Other studies have focused on perturbations of cell organelles or cell-signalling pathways which are traditionally activated in other experimental models of inflammation, fibrosis and carcinogenesis. These assays have been valuable in determining mechanisms of disease and the properties of fibres, i.e. length and free-radical-generating properties, which are important in cell transformation and proliferation (Mossman & Begin, 1989).

The mechanisms of fibre-induced carcinogenicity have been recently reviewed by IARC (1996).

6.3.1 Genotoxicity and interactions with DNA

Table 22 summarizes results of some key *in vitro* genotoxicity studies.

Many studies have been performed to determine whether or not chrysotile and other types of asbestos interact with DNA either directly by physical association or indirectly via the production of reactive oxygen species (ROS), which may be generated primarily by iron-driven redox reactions on the surface of fibres. The latter mechanism may be particularly relevant to the enhanced biological activities of crocidolite and amosite, which contain approximately 26-36% iron, in comparison to chrysotile (generally < 2% iron by weight), in some preparations (Lund & Aust, 1991). The importance of iron in these reactions is illustrated by the observations that the DNA breakage is also observed with ferric citrate (Toyokuni & Sagripanti, 1993), and that reactivity of fibres is inhibited with iron chelators, such as desferrioxamine (Lund & Aust, 1991). Cell-free assays have shown that UICC samples of Canadian chrysotile, amosite and crocidolite cause lipid peroxidation (Weitzman & Weitberg, 1985), presumably

Table 22. In vitro studies on genotoxicity

Species (cell type)	Type of fibres	End-point (change)	Results	Reference
Drosophila (female germ cells)	NIEHS samples of chrysotile, crocidolite, amosite, tremolite	Aneuploidy (+)	Chrysotile and amosite (+) at high dose (25 mg/ml), only chrysotile (+) at low (5 mg/ml) dose. No effects with other types of asbestos.	Osgood & Sterling, 1991
Rat (pleural mesothelial cells)	Canadian chrysotile; UICC crocidolite	Aneuploidy (+); chromosomal aberrations (+)	Chrysotile caused more effects on a weight basis, but crocidolite more effects on a fibre basis. NOEL in 1 of 2 experiments.	Yegles et al., 1993
Rat (pleural mesothelial cells)	Canadian chrysotile	Aneuploidy (+)	NOEL	Jaurand et al., 1986
Rat (pleural mesothelial cells)	UICC chrysotile	Morphologic transformation (+)	Only one dose evaluated.	Paterour et al., 1985
Rat (lung epithelial cells)	NIEHS intermediate chrysotile	Polyploidy (+); chromosomal aberrations (+)	Dose-dependent increases.	Li, 1986
Rat (bone marrow cells)	Indian chrysotile	Chromosomal aberrations (+)	Increase in chromosomal aberrations; decrease in mitotic index of bone marrow cells. Only one dose evaluated	Fatma et al., 1992

Table 22 (contd).

Cell type	Fibre type	Endpoint	Results	Reference
Golden Syrian hamster (embryo cells)	UICC chrysotile; glass fibre 100, 110; amosite; crocidolite; anthophyllite; Benzo(a)pyrene (BP)	Morphologic transformation (+)	Chrysotile caused the strongest effects on a weight basis. No synergistic effects of BP	Mikalsen et al., 1988
Chinese hamster (lung fibroblast)	UICC chrysotile; UICC crocidolite; erionite	Aneuploidy (+); chromosomal aberrations (+)	NOEL, erionite > crocidolite > chrysotile on a fibre basis	Palekar et al., 1987
Chinese hamster (lung fibroblasts)	35 dusts, including UICC and sized UICC chrysotile	Chromosomal aberrations (+)	Chrysotile more active on a weight basis than other types of asbestos. No dose-response. Shorter preparations less active than long fibres.	Koshi et al., 1991
Mouse Balb/3T3 (fibroblasts)	UICC chrysotile; UICC crocidolite TPA[e]	Morphological transformation (+)	With chrysotile, dose-response increases in transformation. Chrysotile and TPA act synergistically.	Lu et al., 1988
Hamster-human hybrid (fibroblasts)	UICC chrysotile	Mutations at HGPRT (-) and S_1 locus (+)	Dose-response mutations at S_1 locus.	Hei et al., 1992
Human (bronchial epithelial cells)	UICC chrysotile A; UICC crocidolite	Chromosomal aberrations (-) binuclei and micronuclei (-,+)	No statistically significant effect of chrysotile on numerical or structural chromosome changes. Dose-dependent (NOEL) in micronuclei and binuclei only at 3 days.	Kodama et al., 1993

Table 22 (contd).

Species (cell type)	Type of fibres	End-point (change)	Results	Reference
Human (lung fibroblasts)	UICC chrysotile A; glass fibres	Mitotic index (-)	Cytological changes with chrysotile indicative of cell death (scattered chromatin observed). No effects of glass fibres.	Verschaeve et al., 1985
Human (lymphocytes)	Chrysotile (USSR); Clinoptilite; Latex	Chromosomal aberrations (+)	Latex and clinoptilite also + at same weight concentration as chrysotile	Korkina et al., 1972
Human female (pleural, mesothelial cells)	UICC chrysotile; UICC crocidolite; UICC amosite	Chromosomal aberrations (+)	Only one concentration evaluated. Numerical and structural alterations with all asbestos types, but no breakage nor polyploidy. Aberrations in 2/4 untreated controls.	Olofsson & Mark, 1989

[a] TPA = 12-O-tetradecanoylphorbol-13-acetate

by catalysing the formation of toxic hydroxyl radicals from hydrogen peroxide, a reaction inhibited by desferrioxamine (Weitzman & Graceffa, 1984; Gulumian & Van Wyk, 1987).

Chrysotile asbestos causes breakage of isolated DNA *in vitro* (Kasai & Nishimura, 1984), but this phenomenon is also observed with ferric citrate (Toyokuni & Sagripanti, 1993) and other chemical systems that generate ROS. Oxidative damage to DNA, as indicated by the formation of 8-hydroxydeoxyguanosine from deoxyguanosine (Leanderson et al., 1988), or calf thymus DNA (Adachi et al., 1992) *in vitro* is more potent with chrysotile in comparison to man-made fibres on an equal weight basis. However, the hydroxyl-radical-producing capacity attributed to this activity may be related more directly to the surface area of the material (Leanderson et al., 1988).

Chrysotile asbestos has been shown to induce chromosomal aberrations (Sincock et al., 1982; Lechner et al., 1985; Jaurand et al., 1986), anaphase abnormalities (Palekar et al., 1987; Pelin et al., 1992; Jaurand et al., 1994), and sister chromatid exchange (Livington et al., 1980; Kaplan et al., 1980) in cultured rodent and human cells.

6.3.2 Cell proliferation

Interactions of chrysotile with the DNA of rodent cells may result in chromosomal or mutational events indicative of the initiation of carcinogenesis or genetic damage associated with cytolysis and cell death. However, cell proliferation, a phenomenon intrinsic to the long promotion and progression phases of the carcinogenic process, may be a more important contributing factor to both cancer and fibrosis. Sustained increases in incorporation of tritiated thymidine have been documented in human embryonic lung fibroblasts after exposure to UICC chrysotile at 10 µg/ml medium, but not at 5 µg/ml (Lemaire et al., 1986b). Moreover, effects were not observed with latex beads or titanium dioxide at up to 10-fold higher concentrations. In hamster tracheal epithelial cells, both UICC chrysotile and crocidolite asbestos caused increases in activity of ornithine decarboxylase (ODC), a rate-limiting enzyme in the biosynthesis of polyamines, which accompanied increases in labelling by tritiated thymidine in these cells (Landesman & Mossman, 1982; Marsh & Mossman, 1988, 1991).

Elevations in ODC activity were also observed with Code 100 fibreglass and long chrysotile (>10 µm) fibres, but to a lesser extent with short chrysotile (<2 µm) (Marsh & Mossman, 1988).

Both rats (Brody & Overby, 1989; McGavran et al., 1990) and mice (McGavran et al., 1990), following a single exposure to approximately 10 mg/m^3 air, exhibited rapid reversible proliferation of epithelial and interstitial cells, as measured by incorporation of tritiated thymidine, which was followed by increased accumulation of alveolar macrophages and localized interstitial fibrosis using morphometric techniques (Chang et al., 1988). In mice, endothelial and smooth muscle cells of arterioles and venules near alveolar duct bifurcations, the site of deposition of asbestos fibres, also incorporate increased levels of tritiated thymidine up to 72 h after initiation of a 5-h exposure to chrysotile (McGavran et al., 1990).

Morphometric analyses of ultrastructural changes in chrysotile-exposed rat lungs have also been used to determine the responses of alveolar type II epithelial cells after inhalation of chrysotile asbestos over a 2-year period (Pinkerton et al., 1990). During this time, type II cell number and volume increased to values more than 4 times those seen in controls. Inhalation of chrysotile over a one-year period resulted in regional differences in the localization and lung burden of fibres, which were proportional to the relative degree of tissue injury at that site (Pinkerton et al., 1986).

The induction of protooncogenes which govern cell division has been compared in cultures of rat pleural mesothelial cells (RPM) and hamster tracheal epithelial cells (HTE) (Heintz et al., 1993). These studies indicated that UICC crocidolite asbestos and UICC chrysotile asbestos cause persistent induction of the protooncogenes c-fos and c-jun in RPM cells in a dosage-dependent fashion. Crocidolite was much more potent than chrysotile in stimulating gene expression of both protooncogenes on a fibre number basis. In HTE cells, only c-fos induction was observed, but patterns of induction by both types of asbestos were similar to those observed in RPM cells. No increases were documented with the use of polystyrene beads or riebeckite.

Effects on Laboratory Mammals and In Vitro Test Systems

6.3.3 Inflammation

Using intratracheal injection (1, 10, 25, 50 or 100 mg of UICC Canadian chrysotile) into the isolated tracheal lobe of the lungs of sheep and following pulmonary lavage, Begin et al. (1986) examined the extracted fluid and cells for evidence of inflammation by differential cell counts and estimations of lactate dehydrogenase (LDH), alkaline phosphatase, β-glucuronidase and levels of fibronectin and procollagen. Only the 100 mg dose produced any changes from control levels, a finding which the authors suggested supported the idea of a "tolerance threshold". Comparing UICC Canadian chrysotile to short Canadian chrysotile and a chrysotile coated with either phosphate or aluminium (intratracheal injection of 100 mg), the UICC chrysotile preparation and the samples of coated chrysotile all produced evidence of similar levels of pulmonary inflammation, but the short chrysotile preparation produced no changes from control values. By administering 100 mg of chrysotile intratracheally at 10-day intervals, Begin et al. (1990) found that normal sheep showed much less evidence of pulmonary inflammation in lavage fluids than those with fibrosis, and the fibre retention was 2.5 times greater when fibrosis was present.

Lemaire et al. (1985) administered, by a single intratracheal injection, 5 mg of either UICC Canadian chrysotile or short fibre preparation (all fibres < 8 μm in length) to rats. Lung morphology was examined at intervals of up to 60 days. The UICC chrysotile produced nodular lesions around the terminal bronchioles with accumulation of inflammatory cells followed by collagen deposition. In contrast, the short fibre preparation produced an accumulation of inflammatory cells but no fibrosis. It was found that standard chrysotile caused an influx of PMN during the first day, which persisted for 7 days. In contrast, the short chrysotile caused only a transient increase in PMN on day 1. Both preparations stimulated an influx of lavageable macrophages, which were frequently binucleate, and frequent mitotic figures were recorded. These studies were extended to include different dose levels and to include attapulgite, xonotlite and aluminium silicate fibres. Intratracheal dose levels were 1, 5 and 10 mg. One month after treatment, UICC Canadian chrysotile and aluminum silicate, which contained long fibres, had produced fibrotic lesions at all doses, while short chrysotile and attapulgite (a short fibre clay material) produced an accumulation of inflammatory cells but no fibrosis. Xonotlite produced only a minimal response.

Pulmonary lavage was used to examine the inflammatory response to chrysotile and amosite dust in rats following short-term inhalation (Donaldson et al., 1988a; Davis et al., 1989). UICC Rhodesian chrysotile produced a rapid increase in both lavageable macrophages and PMN within 2 days of the start of inhalation at a dose level of 10 mg/m^3. Amosite at the same dose had little effect; the chrysotile response was even greater than the early response stimulated by amosite at 50 mg/m^3. By 52 days of study, the 50 mg amosite dose had elicited more macrophages than 10 mg of chrysotile, and by 75 days it had elicited more neutrophils as well. By 75 days, the numbers of macrophages in lavage fluids was falling in both chrysotile and amosite treatments, perhaps because macrophages aggregated around fibre deposits were becoming less susceptible to lavage. In contrast to the findings with asbestos, quartz at a concentration 10 mg/m^3 produced only minimal increases in macrophages and neutrophils during the first 30 days of dusting, but subsequently a massive influx of both cell types occurred and persisted until the end of the study. In this report, levels of LDH and β-glucuronidase in lavage fluids closely mirrored the numbers of lavage cells for all dust types. Donaldson et al. (1990) used the same experimental procedure to examine leucocyte chemotaxis. Following inhalation for up to 75 days of chrysotile, amosite, quartz or titanium dioxide, chemotactic activity towards zymosan-activated serum was found to be reduced with the first 3 dusts. In contrast, chemotaxis of cells lavaged from animals treated with titanium dioxide showed only a small impairment of chemotaxis. After inhalation of chrysotile (10 mg/m^3) for 1 h, cells from BAL exhibited a diminished capacity to secrete superoxide anion, an active oxygen species implicated in bactericidal activity, when incubated with the opsonized zymosan (Petruska et al., 1990).

6.3.4 Cell death and cytotoxicity

Several studies have documented the short-term cytotoxic effects of chrysotile asbestos and other particulates on cells in culture (reviewed in Mossman & Begin, 1989). These studies indicate that geometry and size are important determinants of cytotoxicity in a number of cell types; longer fibres are more potent than short fibres in most of these bioassays (Wright et al., 1986; Mossman & Sesko, 1990).

6.3.5 Liberation of growth factors and other response of cells of the immune system

Macrophages and other cell types of the immune system produce a number of cytokines or growth factors (Rom & Paakko, 1991; Schapira et al., 1991; Perkins et al., 1993), products of arachidonic acid and lipoxygenase metabolism (Kouzan et al., 1985; Dubois et al., 1989), proteolytic enzymes (Donaldson et al., 1988b), neuropeptides (Day et al., 1987), immunomodulation factors (Bozelka et al., 1986), chemotactic factors (Hays et al., 1990), and activated oxygen species (Cantin et al., 1988) after exposure to chrysotile asbestos (reviewed in part by Mossman & Begin, 1989). Whether these substances are important causally to the induction of asbestos-associated disease or in mitigating the disease process is unclear. For example, some of these factors, such as platelet-derived growth factor (PDGF), are also induced after exposure to iron spheres (Schapira et al., 1991) and other innocuous particles used as negative controls. However, such particles are not translocated to the interstitium, while chrysotile fibres are readily translocated (Brody & Overby, 1989).

The initial inflammatory response to inhaled asbestos fibres and subsequent development of fibrosis, and also possible neoplasia, is claimed to be mediated by a number of chemical factors, most of which are produced by pulmonary macrophages that have phagocytosed fibres. Lemaire et al. (1986c) examined the production of fibroblast growth factor (FGF) by pulmonary macrophages from rats given a single intratracheal injection of either 5 or 10 mg of Canadian chrysotile. In control rats, pulmonary macrophages secrete FGF while monocytes from peripheral blood secrete fibroblast growth inhibitory factor (FGIF). Subsequent to asbestos treatment, secretion of FGF by pulmonary macrophages was significantly increased and monocyte production of FGIF was reduced. The stimulation of fibroblast proliferation by alveolar macrophages was further examined by co-culturing macrophages from normal rats and rats treated by a single intratracheal injection of 5 mg of Canadian chrysotile with long fibroblasts (Lemaire et al., 1986d). Macrophages from chrysotile-treated animals caused significantly more fibroblast proliferation than controls. Bonner & Brody (1991) demonstrated that, when rats were exposed for only 3 h to chrysotile at a dose level of 10 mg/m^3, macrophages lavaged one week later stimulated 2-5 times more production of PDGF than controls. However, exposure to iron (50 mg/m^3) caused a similar increase. Cantin et al. (1989) showed that development of asbestosis is associated with increased secretion of plasminogen activator by pulmonary macrophages. In sheep given 100 mg of Canadian chrysotile every 2 weeks by intratracheal injection, some animals developed fibrosis and some did not. Lavaged macrophages from animals developing fibrosis were found to secrete larger amounts of plasminogen activator than those from animals that did not developed fibrosis. Bonner et al. (1993) believe that the combination of retention and translocation, along with release of growth factors and other inflammatory mediators, is responsible for the fibrogenic effects of fibres.

After exposing rats by inhalation to chrysotile or crocidolite asbestos at a dose level of approximately 10 mg/m^3 for up to 91 days, Hartmann et al. (1984a,b) found that the expression of the Ia antigen on macrophages lavaged from crocidolite-treated animals was increased 4-fold in male Fischer-344 rats while chrysotile produced no increase over controls. In female ACI rats, crocidolite produced similar effects but in these animals chrysotile also stimulated an increase in Ia expression at approximately half the level of crocidolite. Significantly greater thymocyte DNA synthesis was induced by supernatants from co-cultures of alveolar macrophages and splenic lymphocytes from asbestos-treated rats than from controls.

An effect on splenocyte mitogenesis by chrysotile treatment was noted by Hannant et al. (1985). In these studies rats were given a 10 mg intraperitoneal injection of Rhodesian chrysotile, quartz or titanium dioxide. After 14 days, splenocytes from animals treated with chrysotile or quartz showed a significant reduction in mitogenic response to phytohaemagglutinin and concanavalin A compared to controls. Titanium dioxide produced no effect. Intraperitoneal injection of chrysotile into mice caused impairment of subsequent production of antibody to the protein antigen.

7. EFFECTS ON HUMANS

Studies reviewed are restricted to those that were considered by the Task Group to be of clear relevance to characterizing the risks associated with exposure to chrysotile. Limitations of particle-to-fibre count conversions on which the exposure estimates in the following studies are based are presented in Chapter 2.

7.1 Occupational exposure

7.1.1 Pneumoconiosis and other non-malignant respiratory effects

The non-malignant lung diseases resulting from exposure to asbestos fibres comprise a somewhat complex mixture of clinical and pathological syndromes not readily definable for epidemiological study. Traditionally, the prime concern has been asbestosis, generally implying a disease associated with diffuse interstitial pulmonary fibrosis accompanied by varying degrees of pleural involvement. More recently, as severe asbestosis has become less frequent clinically, attention has been directed primarily to syndromes reflecting fibrosis of the small and large airways rather than of the lung parenchyma. As a cause of death, the pneumoconioses have never been reliably recorded on death certificates. In investigations of mortality, therefore, all chronic non-malignant respiratory diseases are generally considered as one group. Additionally, mortality studies are generally not sufficient to detect clinically significant morbidity. Equally, in studies of morbidity, the etiological or diagnostic specificity of the usual methods of assessment, i.e. chest radiography, physiological testing and symptom questionnaire, is limited.

Early studies in both the United Kingdom and USA demonstrated an extremely high prevalence of asbestosis among textile workers exposed only to chrysotile at very high dust levels (Dreeson et al., 1938).

Extensive morbidity surveys of chrysotile workers were initiated in the Quebec chrysotile mines and mills in the 1960s (McDonald et al., 1974). These studies included the use by six readers of the then newly developed UICC/Cincinnati (later ILO) radiographic classification of nearly 7000 films, examinations by questionnaire and lung function tests of over 1000 current employees, and detailed assessments of cumulative dust exposure for each man. In the initial survey, there was a fairly systematic relationship between exposure and these measures of response. The authors concluded that exposure to 70-140 mpcm (2-4 mpcf) for a working life of 50 years was associated with a 1% risk of acquiring clinically significant disease.

Based on additional study of radiological changes in 515 men aged 60-69 years (average 64.6 years) who had been employed for at least 20 years (average 42.3 years) at Thetford Mines, the dustier of the two Quebec mining regions, dose–response relationships for small opacities were essentially linear (Liddell et al., 1982). However, any increase in prevalence in small opacities (>1/0 or >2/1) above the level of the intercepts (which were high) only became apparent at an accumulated exposure at age 45 of 1200 f/ml-years, equivalent to an average concentration of about 30 f/ml (Liddell et al., 1982). In contrast to small opacities, pleural thickening was not related to cumulative exposure, although it was more common in men with long service.

Becklake et al. (1979) reported a second study in Quebec of 86 men whose last chest film was taken within 12 months of leaving employment in 1960-1961, and who were examined again in 1972. In 66 men who had been employed for at least two years, there was evidence of an increase in small irregular parenchymal opacities in 8 men (12%) but in none of the 20 men with shorter employment. Increase of pleural thickening was seen in a further 13 (20%) of the 66 men and 4 (20%) of the 20 men.

A dose-related reduction in vital capacity ($p = 0.023$) and expiratory volume ($p < 0.001$) was observed with increasing cumulative exposure (i.e. ≥ 8 f/ml-years) to chrysotile asbestos in miners and millers (stratified random sample of 111 men) in Zimbabwe, exposed for more than 10 years. The relationship between cumulative exposure and radiographic parenchymal category demonstrated a steep increase with each change in category ($p < 0.00001$). Individual estimates of cumulative exposure based on company records of employment history and fibre concentrations (measured and estimated) ranged from 1.1 to

654 fibres/ml-years. Controls were a subset of miners (n=66) with no prior respiratory illness, who were lifelong non-smokers with normal chest X-ray and minimal cumulative exposure to chrysotile asbestos (<8 fibres/ml-years) (Cullen et al., 1991).

A number of other studies of radiographic and functional changes have been conducted in occupational populations exposed primarily to chrysotile, in some cases during mining and milling operations (Rubino et al., 1979a; McDermott et al., 1982; Viallat et al., 1983; Cordier et al., 1984; Enarson et al., 1988), asbestos-cement (Weill et al., 1979; Jones et al., 1989) and asbestos textiles (Berry et al., 1979; Becklake et al., 1980). Results were generally comparable to those already described, the presence of small opacities increasing with cumulative exposure (although with some variability in the shape and steepness of these trends) and pleural changes primarily related to time since initial exposure. As demonstrated in several of these studies, e.g., Becklake et al., 1979; Rubino et al., 1979a; Berry et al., 1979; Viallat et al., 1983, and as well recognized clinically, X-ray changes can develop among workers after exposure ceases, in some cases many years later.

Studies that correlate disease prevalence or symptoms with cumulative exposure can underestimate disease risk due to progression of disease after employment ceases. Although workers were exposed to both chrysotile and crocidolite (the latter being approximately 5% of all asbestos used), results for 379 men employed at least 10 years in the Rochdale asbestos textile plant are informative in this regard (Berry et al., 1979). Exposure estimated from work histories ranged from an average of 2.9 to 14.5 f/ml. Overall, small opacities (>1/0) were recorded in 88/379 (23%) of chest radiographs, with evidence of a gradient seriously confounded by date of first employment and transfer of subjects with suspected asbestosis to less dusty conditions. On the basis of data on incidence, the authors drew conclusions on exposure–response between cumulative exposure and prevalence or incidence of crepitations, possible asbestosis and certified asbestosis - all three depending on clinical opinion and judgement. The authors concluded that possible asbestosis occurs in no more than 1% of men after 40 years of exposure to concentrations between 0.3 and 1.1 f/ml.

Mortality studies of Quebec miners and millers by McDonald et al. (1994) have shown exposure–response relationships for pneumoconiosis-related mortality. Crude rates of 0.23 cases per 1000 man-years were observed for those with cumulative exposures less than 3530 mpcm-years (100 mpcf-years) and a rate of 2.7 cases per 1000 man-years was reported for those with more than 10 590 mpcm-years (> 300 mpcf-years). Dement et al. (1994) also reported mortality due to non-malignant respiratory diseases among chrysotile textile workers. An SMR of 1.88 was observed for those with cumulative exposures less than 2.7 f/ml-years and rose rapidly to 12.78 with cumulative exposures greater than 110 f/ml-years. It was noted that cases of pneumoconioses recorded on death certificates are often verified by pathological diagnosis.

Chest X-ray changes among textile and friction product workers in China were reported by Huang (1990). A total of 824 workers employed for at least 3 years in a chrysotile products factory from the start-up of the factory in 1958 until 1980, with follow-through to September 1982, were studied. Chest X-ray changes compatible with asbestosis were assessed using the Chinese standard system for interpretation of X-rays. Cases were defined as Grade I asbestosis (approximately equivalent to ILO $\geq$1/1). Overall, 277 workers were diagnosed with asbestosis during the follow-up period, corresponding to a period prevalence of 31%. Exposure–response analysis, based on gravimetric data converted to fibre counts, predicted a 1% prevalence of Grade I asbestosis at a cumulative exposure of 22 f/ml-years.

7.1.2 Lung cancer and mesothelioma

It has been suggested that in the absence of pulmonary fibrosis, lung cancer cannot be attributed to asbestos exposure regardless of fibre type; however, there is also evidence to the contrary. For example, in a recent case–control study, there was evidence of a statistically significant increase in risk of lung cancer without radiological signs of fibrosis (Wilkinson et al., 1995). The question remains the subject of active controversy (Hughes & Weill, 1991; Henderson et al., 1997).

Effects on Humans

Results of cohort studies of workers almost exclusively exposed to chrysotile asbestos and considered by the Task Group to be most relevant to this evaluation are summarized in Table 23 and described in section 7.1.2.1. Studies that contribute less to our understanding of the effects of chrysotile, due primarily to concomitant exposure to amphiboles or to limitations of design and reporting, are presented in section 7.1.2.2. Information most relevant to characterization of risk (i.e. exposure–response assessment) is emphasized.

Assessment of exposure response for mesothelioma is complicated in epidemiological studies by factors such as the rarity of the disease, the lack of mortality rates in the populations used as reference and problems in diagnosis and reporting. In many cases, therefore, cruder indicators of risk have been developed, such as absolute numbers of cases and death and ratios of mesothelioma over lung cancers or total deaths. The mesothelioma/lung cancer ratio in particular is highly variable depending on the industry and the nature and intensity of asbestos exposure, in addition to a number of factors not related to asbestos exposure. Data on mesothelioma occurrence in occupational cohorts should, therefore, be cautiously interpreted.

For the studies reviewed here, the number of mesothelioma deaths is reported, together with the percentage over total deaths (Table 23). It should be noted, however, that additional cases of mesothelioma have been reported in workers from the factories included in the studies reported in Table 23 who were not included in the original cohort studies. However, in the absence of information on the numbers of workers at risk, such reports do not contribute to quantification of risk.

1.2.1   Critical occupational cohort studies - chrysotile

a) Mining and milling

Mortality from lung cancer and mesothelioma has been studied extensively in miners and millers of Quebec and in a smaller operation at Balangero in northern Italy.

Table 23. Results of cohort studies of chrysotile-exposed workers[a]

Study	No. of subjects	All causes No. of deaths	All causes SMR	Lung cancer No. of deaths	Lung cancer SMR	Lung cancer 95% CI[b]	Mesothelioma No. of deaths (percentage)	Mean exposure f/ml	Mean exposure f/ml-years	Slope of dose-response[c]
Mining & Milling										
McDonald et al., 1980[d,e,f]	10 939	3291	1.09	230	1.25	[1.09 - 1.42]	8 (0.24%)	ns	90	0.0006
McDonald et al., 1993[d,e,f]	5335	2800	1.07	315	1.39	[1.24 - 1.55]	25 (0.8%)	ns	90	ns
Nicholson et al., 1979[d]	544	178	1.11	28	2.52	[1.68 - 3.65]	1 (0.56%)	ns	ns	0.0017
Piolatto et al., 1990	1094	427	1.49	22	1.1	[0.7 - 1.7]	2 (0.47%)	ns	ns	ns
Asbestos-cement Production										
Thomas et al., 1982	1592	351	1.02	30	0.91	[0.61 - 1.30]	2 (0.57%)	<2	ns	ns
Ohlson & Hogstedt, 1985[f]	1176	220	1.03	9	1.58	0.72 - 3.00	0 (0%)	2	10-20	ns
Gardner et al., 1986	1510	384	0.94	35	0.92	[0.64 - 1.27]	1 (0.26%)	<1	ns	ns
Hughes et al., 1987 (plant 1)[f]	2565	477	0.91	48[k]	1.17	[0.86 - 1.54]	2 (0.42%)	11	40	0.0003
Hughes et al., 1987 (plant 2)[f,g]	2751	ns	ns	70	1.32	[1.03 - 1.66]	1 (ns)	11	19	0.007
Textile Manufacture										
Dement et al., 1994[h,i]	3022	1258	1.28	126	1.97	[1.64 - 2.35]	2 (0.16%)	5-12	32-105	0.02-0.03
McDonald et al., 1983a[f,h]	2543	570	1.27	59[k]	1.99	[1.52 - 2.57]	1 (0.18%)	ns	ns	0.01

Table 23 (contd).

Friction Materials Production								
Newhouse & Sullivan, 1989[j]	8812	ns	ns	84[k]	0.93 [0.74 - 1.16]	3 (ns)	2-5	0.0006
							12	
McDonald et al., 1984[f]	3641	803	1.09	73[k]	1.49 [1.17 - 1.87]	0 (0%)	ns	0.0005
Mixed products								
Szeszenia-Dabrowska et al., 1988	824	285	1.04	24	1.86 [1.19 - 2.77]	0 (0%)	ns	ns
Cheng & Kong, 1992	1172	151	1.16	21	3.15 [1.95 - 4.81]	ns (ns)	ns	ns
Chen et al., 1988	551	156	ns	19[k]	2.34 [1.41 - 3.67]	1 (0.64%)	ns	ns
Zhu & Wang, 1993	5893	496	ns	18	5.3 [2.67 - 7.1]	ns (ns)	ns	ns

[a] ns = not stated
[b] values in square brackets were calculated by Task Group
[c] Increase in relative lung cancer risk for 1 f/ml-year
[d] Partially overlapping studies
[e] McDonald et al. (1993) extends the follow-up of McDonald et al. (1980)
[f] 20+ years since first employment
[g] Only chrysotile-exposed workers; mean exposure refers to both chrysotile and amphibole workers
[h] Partially overlapping studies
[i] Slopes estimated based on regression of SMRs and risk ratios
[j] Only workers employed after 1950; 10+ years since first employment; dose–response from Berry & Newhouse (1983).
[k] Respiratory cancers

EHC 203: Chrysotile Asbestos

In 1966, a cohort of some 11 000 men and 440 women, born between 1891 and 1920, who had worked for one month or more in chrysotile production in Asbestos and Thetford Mines and 400 persons employed in a small mixed asbestos products factory in Asbestos, Canada, was identified. The cohort, which has now been followed up to 1988, was selected from a register compiled of all workers, nearly 30 000, ever known to have been employed in the industry. The factory workers were included because there was frequent and often unrecorded movement between the plant and the mine and mill. Apart from a failure to trace 9% of the cohort, most after less than 12 months' employment before 1930, losses have amounted to well under 1%. The intensity of exposure was estimated for each cohort member by year, based on many thousand midget impinger dust particle counts and, more recently, membrane filter fibre counts.

The most relevant analyses of this cohort are those published by McDonald et al. (1980) and McDonald et al. (1993), and in a preliminary fashion by Liddell (1994). In the first of these reports, where 4463 men had died, the standardized mortality ratio (SMR) for men 20 or more years after first employment, assessed against provincial rates, was 1.09 for all causes and 1.25 for lung cancer. There was no excess mortality for lung cancer in men employed for less than 5 years, but at 5 years and above there were clear excesses. Based on analysis by cumulative exposure up to age 45, there was a linear relationship with lung cancer risk.

In the second paper (McDonald et al., 1993), mortality up to the end of 1988 of the 5351 men who had survived into 1976 (of whom 16 could not be traced and 2827 had died) was followed. In this survivor population, the SMRs 20 or more years after first employment were 1.07 for all causes and 1.39 for lung cancer. The investigators subdivided the men into 10 groups based on cumulative exposure up to age 55. The highest relative risk (3.04) was in the highest exposure group ($\geq$ 35 000 mpcm-years; $\geq$ 1000 mpcf-years), the second highest (1.65) was in the second highest exposure group (14 000 to 35 000 mpcm-years; 400 to 1000 mpcf-years) and the third highest (1.50) was in the third highest exposure group (10 500 to 14 000 mpcm-years; 300 to 400 mpcf-years). In the remaining 7 groups below 10 500 mpcm-years (300 mpcf-years), there was no

Effects on Humans

indication of a trend or pattern of exposure–response with relative risks all being above 1 and averaging 1.27. Similar results were obtained in a heavily exposed subset of the cohort with a long duration of exposure (Nicholson et al., 1979). In the analysis of the large Quebec cohort, the relative increase in risk attributable to chrysotile exposure was lower for ex-smokers than smokers and negligible for smokers of 20 or more cigarettes a day. The authors concluded that the interaction appeared to be less than multiplicative.

The number of deaths attributed to mesothelioma in the Quebec cohort has increased with increasing age and time from first employment more rapidly than total mortality (McDonald et al., 1993). At the end of 1988, when some 75% of the cohort had died, and the youngest survivor was aged 73, in a total of 7312 male deaths, there were 33 suspected cases of mesothelioma, 15 coded to ICD 163 and 18 to a variety of other diagnostic codes. After review of all available evidence, including autopsies in 23 and biopsies in 10, the probability of the diagnosis being correct was assessed by the authors as high in 17, moderate in 11, and low in 5. All 33 cases were pleural but in one of low diagnostic probability, the peritoneum was also affected. Of the 33 cases, 20 were miners or millers from Thetford Mines, 8 were miners or millers from Asbestos, and the remaining five cases were observed among men employed in a small asbestos products factory in Asbestos. The median duration of employment was 36 years (range 2.5 to 49 years). There was no case of mesothelioma among the 4371 members of the cohort (40% of 10 925) employed for less than 2 years, eight cases among those 2396 (22%) employed for 2–10 years, and 25 mesotheliomas among the other 38% of the cohort (4158 men) with at least 10 years of employment. Crude rates of mesothelioma by cumulative exposure were calculated. Rates varied from 0.15 cases per 1000 man-years for those with exposures less than 3500 mpcm-years (100 mpcf-years) to 0.97 cases per 1000 man-years for those with exposure of 10 500 mpcm-years (300 mpcf-years) or more.

The most recent account of mortality among the chrysotile miners and millers of Balangero, Italy, was reported by Piolatto et al. (1990) for a cohort comprising 1094 men employed for at least one year between 1946 and 1987, with exposures estimated individually in fibre-years. Of the total, 36 could not be traced and 427 had died. The

SMR for all causes based on national rates was 1.49, a high figure largely explained by hepatic cirrhosis and accidents. Numbers of deaths from all cancers (n=86) and lung cancer (n=22) were close to expected (76.2 and 19.9) and there was no evidence that the risk for either of these causes was related to duration of exposure, fibre-years of cumulative exposure, or time since first or last exposure. Little information was provided on the basis for the estimates of cumulative exposure. The first fibre counts were taken in 1969. Earlier exposure levels were estimated by simulating working situations occurring at various periods since 1946 in the plant, and fibre counts were measured by PCOM (Rubino et al., 1979b).

The cohort of chrysotile production workers employed at the Balangero mine and mill, studied by Piolatto et al. (1990), was almost exactly one tenth the size of the Quebec cohort. At the end of 1987, when 427 (45%) of the cohort had died, there were two deaths from pleural mesothelioma, both in men employed for more than 20 years, with cumulative exposure estimated respectively at 100-400 and > 400 f/ml years. One diagnosis was confirmed histopathologically, and one was based on radiological findings and examination of pleural fluid. Fibrous tremolite was not detected in samples of chrysotile from this mine, but another fibrous silicate (balangeroite), the biological effects of which are not known, was identified in low proportions by mass (0.2-0.5%). At a comparable stage in the evolution of the Quebec cohort, mesothelioma accounted for 10 out of 4547 deaths, a lower but not dissimilar proportion.

b)   Asbestos-cement production

Numerous studies have been conducted on asbestos-cement workers, but only four, analysing five factories, were of groups exposed almost only to chrysotile. In general, cumulative exposures were low, as were the observed SMRs. In the USA, Hughes et al. (1987) studied two asbestos-cement plants in Louisiana. Observed and expected deaths 20 years from onset of employment were provided according to exposure category. In plant 1, which dealt predominantly with chrysotile, small amounts of amosite were used from the early 1940s until the late 1960s and crocidolite for 10 years beginning in 1962. In plant 2, crocidolite was used continuously in the pipe department located in one building. Chrysotile was only used in the remaining three buildings, and lung cancer and mesothelioma mortality data were supplied for workers (63% of the total) whose only employment assignment was in these buildings. Cohort mortality analyses were conducted for both plant 1 and plant 2 workers 20 or more years after initial employment. There were 22 respiratory cancer deaths among 996 plant 1 employees with more than 6 months of service, which indicated a small non-significant lung cancer risk. However, a corresponding analysis of 42 lung cancer cases among 1414 plant 2 employees with more than 3 months of service and no assignment in the pipe building indicated a substantial lung cancer risk. Two deaths attributed to mesothelioma were reported among cohort members at plant 1 (mean exposure of 40 f/ml-years), while 1 death from mesothelioma was reported among workers at plant 2 (mean exposure of 19 f/ml-years).

Among 1176 Swedish asbestos-cement workers who were estimated to have used >99% chrysotile (Ohlson & Hogstedt, 1985), 11 cases of lung cancer were observed compared to 9 expected (9 observed versus 5.7 expected for those with a 20-year latency). This non-significant increase occurred in a plant with relatively low exposures. In a 10% sample of the work force, all employed for more than 10 years, overall cumulative exposure was 18 f/ml-years. Among the entire cohort, no deaths from mesothelioma were observed. In a study conducted in the United Kingdom (Gardner et al., 1986), the lack of lung cancer increase (35 observed versus 38 expected) can be explained by low cumulative exposures. Since 1970, mean levels were under 1 f/ml throughout the factory and most were under 0.5 f/ml. Higher concentrations of unknown magnitude would have existed prior to 1968. The possibility of low level smoking in the workforce compared to the general population masking lung cancer risks from chrysotile is considered unlikely by the authors. One death from mesothelioma (0.26% of total deaths) was reported among cohort members in this study. A study by Thomas et al. (1982) also did not indicate an excess lung cancer risk (30 observed versus 33.0 expected). Two deaths from mesothelioma (0.57% of all deaths) occurred in this cohort. As with the studies of Ohlson & Hogstedt (1985) and Gardner et al. (1986), the exposures in this plant were very low, the vast majority from 1972 to plant closure being consistently below 1 f/ml.

It must be noted, however, that in most of the cohort studies of asbestos-cement workers, there was no attempt to evaluate the most important confounder of lung cancer, i.e. smoking, or, alternatively, smoking rates were examined only for small subcohorts shortly before the end of follow-up.

(c) Textile manufacture

The health of employees has been studied in any detail in only three asbestos textile plants. These comprise a factory at Rochdale, England, originally studied by Doll (1955) and more recently by Peto et al. (1985), another located in Mannheim, Pennsylvania, USA, studied by McDonald et al. (1983b) and a plant in Charleston, South Carolina, USA. Only the study in South Carolina is considered primarily relevant for assessment of the health effects of chrysotile. Although the SMRs for lung cancer in these plants were broadly equivalent, the rates of mesothelioma varied considerably, which may reflect the greater proportions of amphiboles in the Mannheim and Rochdale cohorts.

The textile workers in the South Carolina plant have been studied in two separate but overlapping cohorts (Dement et al., 1983b; McDonald et al., 1983a; Brown et al., 1994; Dement et al., 1994). The only amphibole used in this plant was approximately one tonne of imported crocidolite from the early 1950s until 1972, plus a very small quantity of amosite for experimental purposes briefly in the late 1950s. The crocidolite yarn was processed at a single location only, so Charleston can be considered an almost pure chrysotile operation. Exposure levels for workers at this plant were estimated by Dementet al. (1983a) using nearly 6000 exposure measurements covering the period 1930–1975 and taking into account changes in plant processes and engineering controls (Table 7). The conversion of past exposures measured in mpcm (mpcf) to f/ml was based on both paired sample data (100 pairs) and concurrent samples (986 samples) by these two methods collected in plant operations during 1968–1971.

The most recent update of the Charleston study by Dement et al. (1994) demonstrated an overall lung cancer SMR of 1.97 (126 observed) and an overall SMR for non-malignant respiratory diseases (ICD 470-478 and 494-519) of 3.11 (69 observed). The data for white males, for which data were more complete, demonstrated an overall lung cancer SMR of 2.34 for those achieving at least 15 years of latency. The risk of lung cancer was found to increase rapidly in relation to cumulative exposure. Data for the entire cohort demonstrated an increase in the lung cancer risk of 2–3% for each fibre/ml-years of cumulative chrysotile exposure. Two mesotheliomas were observed among this cohort and an additional mesothelioma was identified among plant workers, occurred after the study follow-up period. Analyses of an overlapping cohort from the same factory (McDonald et al., 1983a) provided similar results.

It can be seen in Table 23 that the regression line slopes for relative risks of lung cancer in relation to accumulated exposure in the Charleston plant are all some 30 times steeper than those observed in chrysotile mining and cement product manufacture.

(d) Friction materials manufacture

There have been only two cohort studies in which the risks of lung cancer in the manufacture of asbestos friction materials have been examined. One of these was among employees of a plant in Stratford, Connecticut, USA, which used only chrysotile (McDonald et al., 1984). The other was in a large plant in the United Kingdom where, apart from two periods before 1944 when crocidolite was needed for one particular contract, only chrysotile was used (Berry & Newhouse, 1983; Newhouse & Sullivan, 1989).

In the United Kingdom plant, there were no excesses in deaths due to all causes or to lung cancer (Newhouse & Sullivan, 1989). Berry & Newhouse (1983) carried out case–control studies on deaths from lung cancer and gastrointestinal cancer using a detailed assessment based on the work history for each subject and estimated levels of chrysotile exposure. The first fibre counts were taken in 1968. Earlier work practices were simulated using original machinery and appropriate basic materials to estimate historical fibre counts. Fibre counts (both personal and static sampling) were measured by PCOM (Skidmore & Dufficy, 1983) (Table 10). There was no evidence of any exposure–response relationship for either cancer site. For lung cancer, an estimated relative risk of 1.06 for a cumulative exposure of 100 f/ml-years was associated with a 95% confidence interval of 0.6 to 2.0. A total of 13 deaths from mesothelioma (0.54% of all deaths) was observed among this cohort.

The study in Stratford, Connecticut, was complicated by the fact that the high SMR for lung cancer, based on state death rates, was largely explained by mortality among men employed in the plant for less than one year. The exposure–response relationship for lung cancer was described; however, there was in fact no significant relationship between risk and cumulative exposure. No mesotheliomas were observed among the cohort members in this study.

(e) Mixed products manufacture

In a study of 824 workers employed during 1946–1973 in a factory producing various chrysotile products in Lodz, Poland, and followed-up until 1985, there was a significant increase in lung cancer mortality, based on 24 observed and 12.9 expected deaths (SMR 1.86, 95% CI 1.19–2.77). When workers were grouped according to cumulative asbestos dust exposure, the SMR of lung cancer was 1.55 in the group with exposure to up to 50 mg/m^3-years and 3.11 in the group with higher exposure (Szeszenia-Dabrowska et al., 1988). No mesotheliomas were observed among the cohort members in this study.

In a cohort of 1172 workers in Tianjin, China, exposed to chrysotile in the manufacture of asbestos textiles, friction materials and asbestos-cement for at least one year, and followed from January 1972 to December 1987, Cheng & Kong (1992) reported increased risk of mortality from lung cancer (21 observed/6.67 expected; SMR= 3.15; $p<0.05$) and "other" non-malignant respiratory disease (29 observed/11.78 expected; SMR= 2.46; $p<0.05$). The comparison was made with the general population of Tianjin. Based upon employment history and monitoring data collected between 1964 and 1975, estimates of qualitative and quantitative (i.e. low, middle or high;

cumulative exposures of <400, 400–800 or ≥800 mg/m^3-years) exposure to "asbestos dust" were derived for each worker. The Task Group noted that these exposures were extremely high. Analysis of the relative risk of lung cancer according to level, duration or latency since first exposure indicated significant excess risk of mortality at all levels of cumulative exposure (SMRs ranged from 2.71 to 4.85; p <0.01), with "middle" or "high" levels of exposure (p <0.01), with duration of exposure ≥ 15 years (SMRs ranged from 3.02 to 6.67; p <0.01), and with ≥ 20 years latency (SMRs ranged from 2.97 to 3.11; p <0.05). Information on the distribution of workers across industries or movement of workers from one industry to another was not reported.

Chen et al. (1988) reported mortality for 1551 workers in Shanghai, China, producing asbestos textiles, rubber, brake linings, seal material and thermal insulation products between 1958 and 1985. Compared to the population of Shanghai, lung cancer was increased (SMR = 2.28, 14 observed for males; SMR = 2.17, 5 observed for females).

Zhu & Wang (1993) reported significantly increased relative risk (RR= 5.3; 95% CI= 2.6–7.1) and attributable risk (AR= 63.6%; p<0.01) of mortality due to lung cancer between 1972 and 1991 in a cohort of 5893 asbestos workers from eight factories in China (45 974 person-years for men and 39 445 person-years for women) exposed to chrysotile compared to a control group of unexposed workers (number not reported; 122 021 person-years). Quantitative data concerning the level of exposure to chrysotile (or other compounds) were not presented.

(f)   Gas mask manufacture

In a study of a group of women who assembled civilian masks using only chrysotile and a group of women who assembled military masks where crocidolite was used, Acheson et al. (1982) reported one death from mesothelioma among 177 deaths in the former group (0.6%) compared with 5 deaths from mesothelioma among 219 deaths (2.3%) in the latter. The experience of the chrysotile group was thus comparable with frequencies observed both in chrysotile mining and milling and in the manufacture of chrysotile-containing products. The authors noted that the case of mesothelioma occurred in a woman who had transferred to the factory that manufactured crocidolite gas masks.

7.1.2.2 Comparisons of lung cancer exposure-response – critical studies

The slopes of the relationship between cumulative exposure to chrysotile and the relative risk of lung cancer are summarized in Table 23 for those studies that reported this information. These studies all expressed this relationship using the following linear relative risk (RR) model:

$$RR = 1 + B \times E$$

where B is the slope and E is the cumulative exposure to chrysotile asbestos expressed in f/ml-years.

The slopes from the studies of the mining and milling industries (0.0006 to 0.0017), the latter having been estimated on a subset of the cohort on which the former was based, and the friction production industries (0.0005 to 0.0006) are reasonably similar. Hughes et al. (1987) in a study of cement workers (section 7.1.2.1b) reported a similar slope (0.0003) in one plant (plant 1) that only used chrysotile, and a nearly 20-fold higher slope (0.007) among workers only exposed to chrysotile in another plant (plant 2).

The slopes of 0.01 and 0.03 reported for the two studies of the chrysotile-exposed textile workers conducted on overlapping populations, as well as the slope of 0.007 from one of the two plants (plant 2) of cement workers in the study of Hughes et al. (1987), were an order of magnitude greater than those reported for the other cohorts. It should be noted that the two textile cohorts were identified from the same textile facility, but were based on different cohort definitions. Hence, it is not surprising that the slopes from these two studies were similar. The slopes in the studies of chrysotile-exposed textile workers are also remarkably similar to those reported in other studies of textile workers with mixed fibre exposures (Peto, 1980; McDonald et al., 1983b; Peto et al., 1985). This similarity in findings provides some support for the validity of the slopes reported in the chrysotile-exposed textile cohorts.

The reason for the much higher slopes observed in studies of textile workers is unknown, although several possible explanations have been suggested. The first is that these differences might be attributed to errors in the classification of exposures in these studies. Particular concern has been raised about errors in the exposure assessment related to conversions from mpcm (mpcf) to fibres/ml that were performed, particularly in the mining and milling studies (Peto, 1989). Sebastien et al. (1989) conducted a lung burden study specifically designed to examine whether the differences in lung cancer slopes observed in the Charleston chrysotile textile cohort and the Quebec mining industries could be explained by differences in errors in exposure estimates. Lung fibre concentrations were measured in: (a) 32 paired subjects that were matched on duration of exposure and time since last exposure; and (b) 136 subjects stratified on the same time variables. Both analyses indicated that the Quebec/Charleston ratios of chrysotile fibres in the lungs were even higher than the corresponding ratios of estimated exposures. This finding was interpreted by the author as being clearly inconsistent with the hypothesis that exposure misclassification could explain the large discrepancy in the lung exposure–response relationships observed in the two cohorts.

Sebastien et al. (1989) offered a second possible explanation for the differences, which was that observations in the Charleston textile cohort may have been confounded by exposure to mineral oils. Dement et al. (Dement, 1991; Dement et al., 1994) have conducted two nested case–control studies designed to evaluate the potential for confounding by exposure to mineral oils in the Charleston textile cohort. Cases and controls were assigned to a qualitative mineral exposure category as well as asbestos exposure. The relationship between chrysotile exposure and lung cancer risk was observed to be virtually unaffected by control for exposure to mineral oils in these analyses. The authors concluded that confounding by machining fluids was unlikely. It should also be noted that studies of other cohorts of workers exposed to machining fluids (including mineral oils) have failed to detect an increase in lung cancer risk (Tolbert et al., 1992).

Finally, it has been suggested that the higher lung cancer risk observed among textile workers might be explained by differences in fibre size distributions (Dement, 1991; McDonald et al., 1993; Dement et al., 1994). Textile operations have been shown to produce fibres that are longer in length than in mining and other operations using chrysotile asbestos (Dement & Wallingford, 1990). The study of Sebastien et al. (1989) also examined the hypothesis that differences in fibre size distribution could explain the discrepancy in lung cancer exposure–response relationships between the Quebec mining and Charleston textile cohorts. Although the authors concluded that differences in fibre size distributions were an unlikely explanation, it was noted that there was a slightly higher percentage of long chrysotile fibres (> 20.5 µm) in the lungs of workers from the Charleston textile facility than in the Quebec miners.

7.1.2.3   *Other relevant studies*

(a)   Mining and milling

Kogan (1982) reported on the morbidity and mortality of chrysotile miners and millers in the former USSR. Dust exposure levels were reported to be extremely high in the 1950s (over 100 mg/m^3) and were substantially reduced to 3 to 6 mg/m^3 in the 1960s and 1970s. The occurrence of asbestosis was substantially reduced by 1979; SMRs of lung cancer in male miners based on reference rates from a neighbouring city were 3.9 during 1948 to 1967 and 2.9 during 1968-1979. In male millers the corresponding values were 4.3 and 5.8. Corresponding figures for women were: miners, 3.9 and 9.4; millers, 2.9 and 9.7 (observed deaths not reported).

Zou et al. (1990) conducted a retrospective cohort mortality study of 1227 men employed at a chrysotile mine in Laiyuen, Hebei province of China, prior to 1972. Mortality in this cohort was compared with that from 2754 local residents of Laiyuen who had never been exposed to asbestos. Based on follow-up of this cohort from 1972 to 1981, 67 deaths were identified (of which 6 were from lung cancer and 3 from mesothelioma) in the asbestos cohort and 247 deaths in the referent population. The lung cancer rate in the exposed cohort was reported to be significantly greater (p<0.001) than the rate

Effects on Humans

in the referent group. The interpretation of this study is limited by the poor description of the methodology used for standardization and statistical testing.

Cullen & Baloyi (1991) reviewed the X-rays, demographic data, and medical and occupational histories for 51 workers with asbestos-related diseases that had been submitted for compensation to a medical board in Zimbabwe since its independence in 1980. One pathologically confirmed case of mesothelioma and one case that radiologically resembled mesothelioma were identified. These cases were associated with occupational exposures to chrysotile asbestos in the Zimbabwe mines and/or mills.

(b) Asbestos-cement production

In other studies of asbestos-cement workers, there has been greater exposure to commercial amphiboles. A study by Neuberger & Kundi (1990, 1993) showed an increased lung cancer risk (SMR = 1.72), which became a small, non-significant one (SMR = 1.04) after adjustment for individual smoking histories. Two studies, (Finkelstein., 1984; Magnani et al., 1987) showed high lung cancer risks (SMRs = 4.8 and 2.68, respectively), suggesting very heavy exposures. All other asbestos-cement worker studies (Clemmensen & Hjalgrim-Jenson, 1981; Alies-Patin & Valleron., 1985; Raffn et al., 1989; Albin et al., 1990) showed positive results, with SMRs up to 1.8; however, smoking was not controlled for in these studies.

(c) Mixed products manufacture

In several reported studies, workers have been exposed to unspecified forms of asbestos in production of either unspecified or mixed products (see, for example, Berry et al., 1985; Enterline et al., 1987).

Epidemiological data for asbestos-exposed workers in Germany who died between 1977 and 1988 were reported in a proportional mortality study by Rösler et al. (1993), although diagnostic criteria were not clearly specified nor was it possible to clearly separate exposure to chrysotile alone from that to mixed fibre types. Among those exposed mainly to chrysotile (464 deaths), the lung cancer proportional mortality ratio (PMR) was 1.54 (95% CI = 1.16-2.01); 24 deaths (5.2%) were due to pleural mesothelioma and 5 (1.1%) to peritoneal mesothelioma. Mortality for those exposed to both chrysotile and crocidolite (115 deaths) was similar, and there was a higher proportion of deaths (3.5%) due to peritoneal mesothelioma. The PMR for pleural mesothelioma was highest in textile manufacture, followed by insulation, paper, cement and polymers, and was lowest in friction product manufacture. Peritoneal mesotheliomas were reported in textile, insulation and cement manufacture.

A series of 843 mesothelioma cases identified during 1960 to 1990 in the state of Saxony-Anholt, which was formerly part of the German Democratic Republic, was reported by Sturm et al. (1994). According to the authors, asbestos products were primarily made from chrysotile asbestos from the Ural mountains of Russia. Only small amounts of chrysotile from Canada and even smaller quantities of amphiboles from Mozambique or Italy were used in manufacturing. The authors indicated that, out of 812 cases with complete data, 67 were exposed only to chrysotile, 331 were exposed to chrysotile and possibly amphiboles, 279 were exposed to both chrysotile and amphiboles, and 135 were exposed only to amphiboles.

(d) Application and use of products

Cohort studies of populations of workers using only or predominantly chrysotile-containing products in applications such as construction have not been identified. Some relevant information is available, however, from population-based analyses of primarily mesothelioma in application workers exposed generally to mixed fibre types.

Although the odds ratio for lung cancer associated with exposure to "asbestos" has been estimated in many case–control studies, the studies have not been in general able to distinguish between chrysotile and amphibole exposure, and are therefore less informative for the present evaluation (see, for example, Kjuus et al., 1986). In a multisite case–control study from Montreal, Canada, however, exposures to chrysotile and to amphiboles were separated, although exposure to amphiboles was not controlled for in the analysis on exposure to chrysotile (Siemiatycki, 1991). In this study, the occupational history of male cases (aged 35-70) of cancer at 20 sites and of 533 population controls was evaluated by a team of industrial hygienists and chemists to assess exposure to 293 agents. Overall, the lifetime prevalence of exposure to chrysotile was 17%, and that of exposure to amphiboles, 6%. The main occupations involving exposure to chrysotile that were considered were motor vehicle mechanics, welders and flame cutters, and stationary engineers. When lung cancer cases (N=857) were compared with cases of all other types of cancers, the odds ratio (OR) of any exposure to chrysotile was 1.2 (90% CI=1.0–1.5; 175 exposed cases), and that of 10 or more years of exposure with at least 5 years of latency ("substantial exposure") was 1.9 (90% CI 1.1–3.2; 30 exposed cases). Corresponding ORs of exposure to amphiboles were 1.0 and 0.9. The OR of exposure to chrysotile was higher for oat cell carcinoma than for other types of lung cancer. Twelve cases of mesothelioma were included in this study. The OR of any exposure to chrysotile was 4.4 (90% CI=1.6–11.9; 5 exposed cases) and that of substantial exposure was 14.6 (90% CI=3.5–60.5; 2 cases). Corresponding ORs of exposure to amphiboles were 7.2 (90% CI=2.6–19.9; 4 cases) and 51.6 (90% CI=12.3–99.9; 2 cases).

Based on analyses of mortality of workers with mixed exposures to chrysotile and amphiboles in the United Kingdom, by far the greatest proportion of mesotheliomas occurs in users of asbestos-containing products, rather than those involved in their production. In the United Kingdom, all death certificates that mention mesothelioma have been recorded since 1968, and 57 000 workers subject to the 1969 Asbestos Regulation or the 1984 Asbestos (Licensing) Regulations have been followed-up. Analyses of these data have led to the following conclusions:

1. Asbestos exposure caused approximately equal numbers of excess deaths from lung cancer (749 observed, 549 expected) and mesotheliomas (183 deaths) within the occupations covered by the 1969 and 1984 regulations (OPCS/HSE, 1995).

2. Only a few (5%) of British mesothelioma deaths were among workers in regulated occupations (Peto et al., 1995). The majority

of deaths occurred in unregulated occupations in which asbestos-containing products are used, particularly in the construction industry. The risk was particularly high among electricians, plumbers and carpenters as well as among building workers.

Extensive case–control studies of 668 cases of mesothelioma as ascertained through pathologists were conducted by McDonald & McDonald (1980) throughout Canada (1960–1975) and the USA (in 1972). Relative risks were as follows: insulation work, 46.0; asbestos production and manufacture, 6.1; heating trades (other than insulation), 4.4. Four subjects were men who had been employed in Quebec chrysotile mines and three were children of employees; no other subjects had lived in the mining area. In some 12 listed occupations, there was no excess of cases over controls, e.g., garage work, carpentry, building maintenance.

Begin et al. (1992) analysed 120 successful claims for pleural mesothelioma submitted to the Quebec Workman's Compensation Board during 1967–1990. Of these, 49 cases occurred among workers in the mining and milling industry, 50 in the manufacturing and industrial application sector and 21 in other types of industry. The miners and millers were thought to be primarily exposed to chrysotile, while the rest were believed to be exposed to mixtures of amphiboles and chrysotile. The numbers of cases ascertained by Begin et al. via the compensation system were consistent with the numbers of incident mesotheliomas observed in miners and millers but grossly underestimated the recorded frequency of mesothelioma in the other industrial sectors (McDonald & McDonald, 1993).

In other large population-based case–control studies of mesothelioma (see, for example, Bignon & Brochard, 1995), it was not possible to separate the effect of chrysotile from that of amphiboles.

Attempts have been made by three groups of investigators to assess the contribution of chrysotile to mesothelioma risk by considering the duration of its use compared with other fibres. These analyses were based, in part, on models for the risk of mesothelioma associated with exposure to various forms of asbestos, which have been widely used by regulatory agencies in the USA, such as the Consumer Product Safety Commission (1987), the Environmental Protection Agency (1986) and the Occupational Safety and Health Administration (1986). Formulae for these models are similar (see, for example, the HEI report) and will not be described here in detail. The analyses include studies of insulation workers (Nicholson & Landrigan, 1994) and railroad machinists in the USA (Mancuso, 1988), and cement workers in Denmark (Raffn et al., 1989). Although the authors of these studies suggest the occurrence of mesothelioma prior to the widespread introduction of amphiboles into industries, there is unresolved controversy about the reliability of the data on which these conclusions are based.

Motor mechanics who repair asbestos-containing brakes and clutches can be exposed to chrysotile, as this is by far the predominant fibre used in this application. Exposures can occur during removal of wear debris from brake and clutch assemblies and during grinding of new linings (Rohl et al., 1976; Rodelsperger et al., 1986). Cases of mesothelioma have been reported among brake mechanics (Langer & McCaughey, 1982; Woitowitz & Rodelsperger, 1991; Woitowitz & Rodelsperger, 1992).

In two case–control studies of mesotheliomas, there was no excess risk among garage workers or mechanics (Teta et al., 1983; Woitowitz & Rodelsperger, 1994). In the latter study, there were two control groups; one was based on hospital cases undergoing lung resection, in most instances because of lung cancer, and the other was from the general population. The authors noted that confounding due to asbestos exposure in other occupations limited their ability to detect mesothelioma risks among car mechanics.

The proportional mortality for mesothelioma among British motor mechanics was reported to be lower than the national average (PMR = 0.40) (OPCS/HSE, 1995). The extent to which all motor mechanics were exposed to friction products was not defined.

7.1.3 *Other malignant diseases*

Results of cohort studies of workers almost exclusively exposed to chrysotile asbestos and considered by the Task Group to be most relevant to this evaluation are summarised in Table 23 and described in section 7.1.3.1. Studies that contribute less to our understanding of the effects of chrysotile, due primarily to concomitant exposure to amphiboles or to limitations of design and reporting, are presented in section 7.1.3.2.

7.1.3.1 Critical occupational cohort studies involving chrysotile

There has been considerable unresolved controversy regarding the possible carcinogenic effect of asbestos on the larynx, kidney and gastrointestinal tract. Moreover, there is little evidence that permits an assessment of chrysotile, in particular, as a risk factor for these cancers. In four of the cohorts exposed almost exclusively to chrysotile, data were presented on SMRs for laryngeal cancer (Hughes et al., 1987; Piolatto et al., 1990; McDonald et al., 1993; Dement et al., 1994). Non-significant excesses were observed in some of the studies. It is not possible to draw conclusions about the association with laryngeal cancer because the data are too sparse and because confounding may play an important role in creating associations. Where examined, laryngeal cancer was strongly associated with cigarette smoking (McDonald et al., 1993) and alcohol consumption (Piolatto et al., 1990).

Owing to the rarity of kidney cancer, cohort studies have limited statistical power to detect even moderate increases of kidney cancer. There was no overall excess of kidney cancer in the cohort of miners and millers followed by McDonald et al. (1993), although some increases occurred in subgroups stratified by mine and exposure; however, the number of cases precludes meaningful interpretation. In the study in asbestos-cement production workers, in which the SMR for kidney cancer in plant 1 (chrysotile) was 2.25, based on only four cases, the SMR for lung cancer was 1.17 (Hughes et al., 1987). No other data on kidney cancer risks were presented for the other cohorts of chrysotile workers.

In predominantly "chrysotile"-exposed cohorts, there is no consistent evidence of excess mortality from stomach or colorectal cancer. In the analysis of mortality in the Quebec cohort up to 1989 (McDonald et al., 1993), the SMR for gastric cancer was elevated in

Effects on Humans

the highest exposure category (SMR = 1.39); the corresponding SMR for lung cancer was 1.85. Overall, there was no systematic relationship with exposure.

7.1.3.2 Other relevant studies

Most case–control studies have investigated the association between exposure to unspecified or several forms of "asbestos" and various cancers (see, for example, Bravo et al., 1988; Parnes, 1990; Jakobsson et al., 1994). In the multisite case–control study conducted in Montreal (see section 7.1.2.3d), 177 cases of kidney cancer were included (Siemiatycki, 1991). The OR of any exposure to chrysotile was 1.2 (90% CI=0.9–1.7; 31 exposed cases), and that of substantial exposure was 1.8 (90% CI=0.9–3.7; 6 cases). Corresponding ORs of exposure to amphiboles were 0.7 (8 cases) and 0.8 (1 case).

In this study, a total of 251 stomach, 497 colon and 257 rectal cancer cases were included (Siemiatycki, 1991). The ORs for any and substantial exposure to chrysotile were 1.3 and 0.7 for stomach cancer, 1.0 and 1.6 (90% CI=1.0–2.5) for colon cancer, and 0.7 and 0.5 for rectal cancer. Exposure to amphiboles was not associated with a significant increase in risk of any of these cancers.

7.2 Non-occupational exposure

Data available on incidence or mortality in populations exposed in the vicinity of sources of chrysotile since Environmental Health Criteria 53 was published have not been identified. In studies reviewed at that time, increases in lung cancer were not observed in four limited ecological epidemiological studies of populations in the vicinity of natural or anthropogenic sources of chrysotile (including the chrysotile mines and mills in Quebec) (IPCS, 1986).

Data available on incidence or mortality in household contacts of asbestos workers were reviewed in Environmental Health Criteria 53. In several case–control studies reviewed therein, there were more mesothelioma cases with household exposure than in controls, after exclusion of occupation. However for most of these investigations, it is not possible to distinguish the form of asbestos to which household contacts were exposed on the basis of information included in the published reports.

Available data on effects of exposure to chrysotile asbestos (specifically) in the general environment are restricted to those in populations exposed to relatively high concentrations of chrysotile asbestos in drinking-water, particularly from serpentine deposits or asbestos-cement pipe. These include ecological studies of populations in Connecticut, Florida, California, Utah and Quebec, and a case–control study in Puget Sound, Washington, USA, reviewed in Environmental Health Criteria 53. On the basis of these studies, it was concluded that there was little convincing evidence of an association between asbestos in public water supplies and cancer induction. More recent identified studies do not contribute additionally to our understanding of health risks associated with exposure to chrysotile in drinking-water.

8. ENVIRONMENTAL FATE AND EFFECTS ON BIOTA

8.1 Environmental transport and distribution

Soils developed on chrysotile-bearing serpentinitic rocks exist in some areas of the world. Brooks (1987) and Roberts & Proctor (1993) have shown that this rock type forms very poor soils and gives rise to unique plant communities. Natural distribution of chrysotile has only become an issue in the last 25 years or so.

Because of their small size, chrysotile fibres may be transported from their place of origin by wind and water. Wind is the primary medium of transport, and, in areas where chrysotile is abundant, large concentrations have been observed in rain and snow run-off (Hallenbeck et al., 1977; Hesse et al., 1977; Bacon et al., 1986). There is contradictory evidence concerning an increase in global concentrations. Cossette et al. (1986) suggested that the global distribution, estimated by chrysotile content in ice core deposits, has been relatively constant. This is in contrast to findings by Bowes et al. (1977), which suggested increases in asbestos deposits in the Greenland ice core samples from the mid-1750s to the present. The mobility of fibres from sites of asbestos-bearing strata is often due to sparse vegetation cover because of adverse physical and chemical conditions not conducive to plant growth.

The management of sediments deposited during flooding by streams draining asbestos- bearing materials appears to be one of the great concerns in relation to environmental exposure. The large water supply system in the California aqueduct is contaminated by run-off containing chrysotile (Hayward, 1984; Jones & McGuire, 1987).

8.1.1 Chrysotile fibres in water

Lake and stream data have been reviewed by Schreier (1989), and chrysotile concentrations are highly variable, depending on proximity to source areas and river flow regime. Concentrations of 1×10^6 to 1×10^8 f/litre are typical in most rivers draining serpentinitic rocks but concentrations of up to 1×10^{13} f/litre have been reported by Schreier (1987) in a stream draining asbestos-bearing bedrock. There are significant seasonal fluctuations in concentrations in most streams and the fibres may remain in suspension for long periods of time.

Chrysotile is very stable in alkaline water but magnesium leaching occurs from the fibre structure under acidic conditions. Many rivers have acidic conditions and chrysotile's surface charge changes from positive in alkaline conditions to negative under acidic conditions (due to the loss of Mg^{2+} from surface brucite layers). In addition, suspended chrysotile fibres may adsorb organic materials, which eventually cover the entire fibre surface (Bales & Morgan, 1985).

8.1.2 Chrysotile fibres in soils

In the absence of organic material, which when present forms organic acids, chrysotile fibres are fairly resistant to alteration. However, in acid soil environments magnesium and trace metals are released and their concentrations locally increased, whereupon they are selectively taken up by plants or soil biota, e.g., by earthworms (Schreier & Timmenga, 1986). Fibres exposed to surface processes will be affected by acid rain and are likely to be transformed. Most attention has been given to the release of trace metals under acidic weathering conditions (Schreier et al., 1987a; Gasser et al., 1995). However, most studies have focussed primarily on the non-fibrous serpentine minerals. While there is evidence of deficiencies and adverse effects on plants and biota, little research has been conducted on the fibre constituents.

8.2 Effects on biota

While the fibre size and geometry appear to be the main issues for human health, the bulk and trace metal chemistry have been identified as factors and agents detrimental to plant growth (Brooks, 1987; Roberts & Proctor, 1993). The chemical impact (little calcium, excess magnesium, chromium, nickel, cobalt) has been studied in many places under the rubric term serpentinitic rock or soil materials, but rarely has chrysotile been identified as the key component mineral.

8.2.1 Impact on plants

The plants most frequently found in serpentinitic environments have been characterized by Brooks (1987) as belonging to insula (neoendemism) and depleted taxa (paleoendemism). Almost all plants on chrysotile-enriched soils show stress symptoms, such as reduced growth, lower frequency, low diversity and slight discoloration. Many serpentine-endemic species have been identified, and coniferous trees appear to be more tolerant to such soils than broadleaf species.

There is great internal variability within sites but moisture, magnesium, low calcium:magnesium ratios, excessive nickel and cobalt, and deficiencies in molybdenum, calcium, phosphorus and nitrogen have all been cited as key factors responsible for poor plant growth. Since many of these factors interact, it is impossible to single out any one of them as the prime factor in limiting vegetation growth. Morphological responses to these adverse conditions are: xeromorphic foliage with different coloration; reduction in size leading to shrubby, stunted plagiotropic appearance; and the development of an extensive root system. Chemical responses are exclusion or restriction of some cations, excess metal uptake and metal storage in different compartments of the plants. There is no universal response by plants to these adverse conditions (Brooks, 1987).

Physical stress results because most of the soils on serpentinitic bedrock are shallow and stoney, leading to poor water-holding capacity. All dark coloured serpentinites exhibit elevated diurnal temperature fluctuations. The moisture stress might be responsible for greater root development, and often such soils are prone to instability. No investigation has thus far been made to determine if the physical properties of fibres are relevant to hazards to plant roots and whether these fibres penetrate into the plant cell walls. In addition, no evidence has so far been provided to suggest that roots are injured when expanding into fibre-rich soils.

The chemical stress is either exerted by excessive concentrations of some elements or serious deficiencies of metals or nutrients. Calcium deficiencies have often been cited as one of the key indicators of stress, but excess metals are likely to be more significant. Most chrysotile-rich soils have neutral to alkaline pH, which reduces metal solubility. Metal accumulation by plants is a topic of interest, and Brooks (1987) proposed the term "hyper-accumulators" for plants that grow on asbestos-rich soils and are enriched in nickel to levels far beyond those found in the soil (Wither & Brooks, 1977; Brooks, 1987).

The use of seeds and plants native to serpentinitic sites is desirable for reclaiming chrysotile-contaminated sites. In addition, native plants on serpentinites do not grow vigorously and do not always respond to amendments (Brooks, 1987; Roberts & Proctor, 1993). Tree seedlings invariably have the greatest difficulties surviving the first year after planting. Almost all plants show stress symptoms and fertilizer amendments are necessary to maintain continuous vegetation cover.

8.2.2 Impact on terrestrial life-forms

Few studies have examined the effect of chrysotile on soil animals. There is a general reduction in soil animals in all such soils, which is not surprising given the low organic matter content and adverse plant growing conditions.

Earthworms are known to tolerate and accumulate trace metals but, in the presence of chrysotile fibres, *Lumbricus rebellus* showed reduced survival (Schreier & Timmenga, 1986) after introduction into chrysotile-rich floodplain sediments. Mortality was attributed to the combined effect of exposure to elevated levels of nickel and magnesium (body burdens were 2-10 times higher in exposed animals relative to controls), as well as the abrasive nature of the fibres.

Termites move large quantities of materials from great depths and, in studies of Zimbabwean serpentinites, Wild (1975) and Brooks (1987) showed increases in pH and levels of nickel, calcium and magnesium in the mounds. The increase in pH might be responsible for reducing the metal toxicity, but the termite soldiers, which consume more mineral materials, were found to have higher nickel and chromium accumulation than termites of higher social orders, which

Environmental Fate and Effects on Biota

consume different food sources provided to them by the soldiers. The termite mounds were found to be fireproof.

Information on microorganisms is also very limited. There are fewer nitrogen fixers in chrysotile-enriched soils (White, 1967; Proctor & Woodall, 1975) and fewer microorganisms (Ritter-Studnicka, 1970). Fungal populations and heterotrophic bacteria are significantly reduced (Bordeleau et al., 1977). At the same time, populations of facultative heterotrophic and autotrophic bacteria are increased. It is unclear what the causes are for these differences. The lack of organic matter, moisture deficiencies, nutrient imbalances and metal toxicities have all been claimed to be responsible for the lack of soil microorganisms. Trace metals, such as nickel, have been found to inhibit the growth of eubacteria, actinomycetes, cyanobacteria, yeasts, filamentous fungi, protozoa and algae (Babich & Stotzky, 1983). In contrast, Deom (1989) showed that mycorrhizal fungi were not adversely affected and were fully functioning in chrysotile-rich soils in central British Columbia, Canada.

Ingested soil plays a significant part in grazing animals. As shown by Thornton (1981), up to 15% of the dry matter intake in sheep and 10% in grazing cattle can be soil. He also suggested that there is a good relationship between metal levels in the soil and those found in the blood of the grazing animals. This was confirmed in cattle grazing in fields affected by chrysotile from flooding events (Schreier et al., 1986). Significant increases in nickel and magnesium were observed in the blood of the animals at the time they were grazing on such fields. Unfortunately the animal population was too small and genetically too diverse to be used for a long-term study.

8.2.3 Impact on aquatic biota

The effect of asbestos fibres on aquatic biota has not been investigated in any detail.

Belanger et al. (1986a, 1987) showed that siphoning activity was significantly reduced, and that growth and reproduction were altered in juvenile *Corbicula fluminea* (Asiatic clam) when exposed to chrysotile fibres. Siphoning activity was reduced by about 20% in juvenile clams exposed to 10^2 to 10^8 f/litre for 30 days; shell growth was significantly reduced at concentrations in the range of 10^4 to 10^8 f/litre (Belanger et al., 1986b). Clams were reported by Belanger et al. (1987) to accumulate chrysotile to a greater degree than any previously tested aquatic organism. Whole-body burdens of clams exposed to 10^8 f/litre for 30 days were nearly 10^3 f/mg (dry weight), while field-collected clams, exposed throughout their lifetime (2-3 years) to about 10^9 chrysotile f/litre accumulated as much as 6.5×10^8 f/mg (dry weight). Graney et al. (1983) reported that these clams also accumulated trace metals.

Lauth & Schurr (1983, 1984) suggested that positively charged chrysotile fibres will attach to planktonic cells, inhibiting their swimming capacity and thus removing a potentially important food source from the water column.

Several studies have been conducted on the effect of chrysotile on fish. Behavioural and histopathological aberrations (a few tumour swellings) were reported in larvae of coho salmon (*Oncorhynchus kisutch*) when larvae were reared in chrysotile-rich water at concentrations of 3×10^6 f/litre for up to 86 days (Belanger et al., 1986c). Growth of larvae of juvenile Japanese medaka (*Oryzias latipes*) was significantly reduced at concentrations of 10^6 to 10^8 f/litre in a 13-week exposure study, and 100% mortality occurred at 10^{10} f/litre after 56 days of exposure. Spawning frequency was 33% higher in control populations of medaka compared with those exposed to 10^4 to 10^8 chrysotile f/litre. After exposure for 3 months to 10^8 f/litre, chrysotile was observed to accumulate in the fish tissue at a concentration of nearly 500 f/mg dry weight (Belanger et al., 1990). Mesothelioma has been reported in fish but no reference was made to asbestos exposure (Herman, 1985).

Trace metal uptake in native fish, exposed to very high chrysotile concentrations in a stream, were reported by Schreier et al. (1987b). These fish did not show any evidence of unusual growth but recorded significant levels of nickel in the epiaxial muscle tissue. In contrast, rainbow trout introduced into a serpentinitic lake with chrysotile concentrations of 2 to 100×10^6 f/litre did not show any adverse effect

5 years after introduction (H. Schreier, 1995, personal communication to the IPCS).

Belanger et al. (1987) have suggested that a specific species of clam, *Corbicula*, may be useful as a biomonitor for chrysotile asbestos in public water supplies.

The impact of chrysotile/serpentine presence and degradation on the environment is difficult to gauge. Observed perturbations are many but their long-term impact is virtually unknown.

9. EVALUATION OF HEALTH RISKS OF EXPOSURE TO CHRYSOTILE ASBESTOS

9.1 Introduction

A previous evaluation by an IPCS Task Group (IPCS, 1986) addressed all types of asbestos, including chrysotile. At that time, it was concluded that: "The risk of mesothelioma in chrysotile-exposed workers is less than that in workers exposed to crocidolite or amosite".

In this monograph (EHC 203), the evaluation is focussed, to the extent possible, on data relevant to assessment of the health risks of exposure to chrysotile, although it should be noted that commercial chrysotile may contain a small proportion of amphiboles, some of which may be fibrous. This was considered appropriate in view of the fact that since the publication in 1986 of the Environmental Health Criteria 53, the use of crocidolite and more recently, amosite, has been largely discontinued. Moreover, the pattern of use of chrysotile asbestos in many countries has changed somewhat, with the asbestos-cement industry being by far the largest user worldwide, accounting for some 85% of all use. Although declining in the North American and Western European markets, asbestos-cement product manufacturing continues to grow in areas including South America, South-East Asia, the eastern Mediterranean region and eastern Europe.

Other chrysotile products include friction products, gaskets and asbestos paper. Production of shipboard and building insulation, roofing and, particularly, flooring felts, and other flooring materials, such as vinyl asbestos tiles, has declined considerably, with some of them disappearing from the market place. Friable chrysotile- and/or amphibole-containing materials in building construction have been phased out in many countries. It should be noted, however, that there are large quantities of these materials still in place in buildings, which will continue to give rise to exposure to both chrysotile and the amphiboles during maintenance, removal or demolition. Chrysotile has been used in hundreds (or even thousands) of products that have entered global commerce. These existing products may also give rise to exposure.

This evaluation is based on studies which the Task Group considered contribute to our understanding of the health risks associated with exposure to chrysotile.

Past uncontrolled mixed exposure to chrysotile and amphiboles has caused considerable disease and mortality in Europe and North America. Moreover, historical experience to mixed fibre types in European countries has clearly indicated that a larger proportion of mesotheliomas occurs in the construction trades than in production. Far larger quantities of chrysotile than of other types of asbestos were used in most construction applications. Epidemiological studies that contribute to our understanding of the health effects of chrysotile conducted to date and reviewed in this monograph have been on populations mainly in the mining or manufacturing sectors and not in construction or other user industries. This should be borne in mind when considering potential risks associated with exposure to chrysotile.

9.2 Exposure

Fibre concentrations reported below are for fibres longer than 5 µm.

9.2.1 Occupational exposure

2.1.1 Production

Exposure is dependent upon such factors as the extent of control, the nature of the material being manipulated and work practices. Based on data available to the Task Group, mainly from North America, Europe and Japan, workplace exposure in the early 1930s was very high in most sectors of the industry for which data are available. Levels dropped considerably between the 1930s and the late 1970s and have continued declining substantially to the present day, owing to the introduction of controls. In the mining and milling industries in Quebec, Canada, the average concentration of fibres in air often exceeded 20 fibres/ml (f/ml) in the 1970s and is now less than 1 f/ml. In the production of asbestos-cement, mean concentrations in the 1970s were typically below about 1 f/ml. Mean concentrations of 0.05

to 0.45 f/ml were reported in Japan in 1992. In asbestos textile manufacture, mean concentrations between 2.6 and 12.8 f/ml in the period between 1970 and 1975 and 0.1 to 0.2 f/ml in the period 1984-1986 were reported in Japan. Trends have been similar in the production of friction materials. Based on data available from Japan, mean concentrations of 10 to 35 f/ml were reported in production during 1970 to 1975, while levels in 1984 to 1986 were 0.2 to 5.5 f/ml. In a plant in the United Kingdom at which a large mortality study was conducted, concentrations were above 20 f/ml before 1931 and generally below 1 f/ml during 1970-1979.

Only limited data on concentrations of chrysotile in occupational environments in countries other than the USA, Europe and Japan were available to the Task Group. The data above on historical levels in uncontrolled conditions and additional information on gravimetric concentrations to which workers are exposed in product manufacture in China indicate that concentrations may be very high (up to 100 f/ml) in production facilities without adequate dust control. In a recent survey of chrysotile mills in India, average concentrations of 2 to 13 f/ml were reported.

9.2.1.2 Use

Few data on concentrations of fibres associated with the installation and use of chrysotile-containing products were available to the Task Group, although this is easily the most likely place for workers to be exposed. During maintenance of vehicles, peak concentrations of 16 fibres/ml were reported in the 1970s in the USA. Practically all measured levels after 1987 were less than 0.2 f/ml, due to introduction of controls. Time-weighted average exposure during passenger vehicle repair reported in the 1980s was less than 0.05 f/ml. However, with no controls, blowing off debris from drums results in short-term high concentrations of dust.

Data on concentrations of airborne fibres associated with manipulation of asbestos-cement products available to the Task Group were sparse. In a South African workshop where asbestos-cement sheets were cut into components for insulation, mean concentrations were 1.9 f/ml for assembling, 5.7 f/ml for sweeping, 8.6 f/ml for drilling and 27 f/ml for sanding. Following clean-up and introduction of controls, levels were 0.5 to 1.7 f/ml.

There is potential for widespread exposure of maintenance personnel to mixed asbestos fibre types due to the large quantities of friable asbestos materials still in place. In buildings where there are control plans, personal exposure of building maintenance personnel in the USA, expressed as 8-h time-weighted averages, was between 0.002 and 0.02 f/ml. These values are the same order of magnitude as exposures reported during telecommunication switch work (0.009 f/ml) and above-ceiling work (0.037 f/ml), although higher concentrations have been reported in utility space work (0.5 f/ml). Concentrations may be considerably higher where control plans have not been introduced. For example, in one case, short-term episodic concentrations ranged from 1.6 f/ml during sweeping to 15.5 f/ml during cleaning (dusting off) of library books in a building with a very friable chrysotile-containing surface formulation. Most other values, presented as 8-h time-weighted averages, are about two orders of magnitude less.

Although few data on exposures among users of asbestos-containing products in industries such as construction were identified, available data clearly demonstrate the need for appropriate engineering controls and work practices for minimizing exposures to chrysotile both in production and use. It should be noted that construction and demolition operations present special control problems.

9.2.2 General population exposure

Sources of chrysotile in ambient air are both natural and anthropogenic. Most airborne fibres in the general environment are short (< 5 µm).

Few recent data on concentrations of chrysotile in air in the vicinity of point sources have been identified. Concentrations around the Shibani chrysotile mine in Zimbabwe ranged from below the limit of detection of the method (<0.01 f/ml) to 0.02 f/ml (fibres longer than 5 µm).

Based on surveys conducted before 1986, concentrations (fibres > 5 μm in length) in outdoor air measured in five countries (Austria, Canada, Germany, South Africa and USA) ranged between 0.0001 and about 0.01 f/ml, with levels in most samples being less than 0.001 f/ml. Means or medians were between 0.00005 and 0.02 f/ml, based on more recent determinations in seven countries (Canada, Italy, Japan, Slovak Republic, Switzerland, United Kingdom and USA).

Fibre concentrations in public buildings during normal use where there is no extensive repair or renovation are within the range of those measured in ambient air, even where friable asbestos-containing materials were extensively used. Concentrations (fibres > 5 μm in length) in buildings in Germany and Canada reported before 1986 were generally less than 0.002 f/ml. In more recent surveys in five countries (Belgium, Canada, Slovak Republic, United Kingdom and USA) mean values were between 0.00005 and 0.0045 f/ml. Only 0.67% of chrysotile fibres were longer than 5 μm.

9.3 Health effects

9.3.1 Occupational exposure

Adverse health effects associated with occupational exposure to chrysotile are fibrosis (asbestosis), lung cancer and mesothelioma. These effects have also been observed in animals exposed to chrysotile by inhalation and other routes of administration. Based on available data in miners and millers, there is an interaction between tobacco smoke and chrysotile in the induction of lung cancer which appears to be less than multiplicative. Epidemiological evidence that chrysotile asbestos is associated with an increased risk of cancer at other sites is inconclusive.

Emphasis in this evaluation is on those studies that contribute to our understanding of the health risks associated with exposure to chrysotile, especially those that characterize at least to some extent, the exposure–response relationship. It should be noted, however, that exposure–response relationships have relied upon reconstruction of historical exposures. This is often problematic, due to lack of historical exposure measurements, and changes in measurement methods that have required use of conversion factors which are highly variable. Moreover, there are wide variations in exposure characteristics, including fibre size distributions, which are not well characterized in traditional measures of exposure.

The Task Group noted that there is an exposure–response relationship for all chrysotile-related diseases. Reduction of exposure through introduction of control measures should significantly reduce risks. Construction and demolition operations may present special control problems.

9.3.1.1 Fibrosis

The non-malignant lung diseases associated with exposure to chrysotile comprise a somewhat complex mixture of clinical and pathological syndromes not readily definable for epidemiological study. The prime concern has been asbestosis, generally implying a disease associated with diffuse interstitial pulmonary fibrosis accompanied by varying degrees of pleural involvement.

Studies of workers exposed to chrysotile asbestos in different sectors have broadly demonstrated exposure–response relationships for chrysotile-induced asbestosis, in so far as increasing levels of exposure have produced increases in the incidence and severity of disease. However, there are difficulties in defining this relationship, due to factors such as uncertainties in diagnosis, and the possibility of disease progression on cessation of exposure.

Furthermore, some variations in risk estimates are evident among the available studies. The reason for the variations is not entirely clear, but may relate to uncertainties in exposure estimates, airborne fibre size distributions in the various industry sectors and statistical models. Asbestotic changes are common following prolonged exposures of 5 to 20 f/ml. The risk at lower exposure levels is not known but the Task Group found no reason to doubt that, although there may be subclinical changes induced by chrysotile at levels of occupational exposure under well-controlled conditions, even if fibrotic changes in the lungs occur, they are unlikely to progress to the point of clinical manifestation.

9.3.1.2 Lung cancer

Exposure–response relationships for lung cancer have been estimated for chrysotile mining and milling operations and for production of chrysotile asbestos textiles, asbestos-cement products and asbestos friction products. Risks increased with increasing exposure. The slopes of the linear dose–response relationships (expressed as the increase in the lung cancer relative risk per unit of cumulative exposure (fibre/ml-years)) were all positive (although some not signficantly) but varied widely. Textiles produce the highest risk (slopes 0.01 to 0.03). Risks for production of cement products (slopes 0.0003-0.007), friction materials (slopes 0.0005-0.0006) and chrysotile mining (0.0006-0.0017) are lower.

The relative risks of lung cancer in the textile manufacturing sector in relation to estimated cumulative exposure are, therefore, some 10 to 30 times greater than those observed in chrysotile mining. The reasons for this variation in risk are not clear.

9.3.1.3 Mesothelioma

Estimation of the risk of mesothelioma is complicated in epidemiological studies by factors such as the rarity of the disease, the lack of mortality rates in the populations used as reference, and problems in diagnosis and reporting. In many cases, therefore, risks have not been calculated, and cruder indicators have been used, such as absolute numbers of cases and death and ratios of mesothelioma over lung cancers or total deaths.

Based on data reviewed in this monograph, the largest number of mesotheliomas has occurred in the chrysotile mining and milling sector. All of the observed 38 cases were pleural with the exception of one of low diagnostic probability, which was pleuro-peritoneal. None occurred in workers exposed for less than 2 years. There was a clear dose–response relationship, with crude rates of mesotheliomas (cases/1000 person-years) ranging from 0.15 for those with cumulative exposure less than 3500 mpcm (< 100 mpcf-years) to 0.97 for those with exposures of 10 500 mpcm (300 mpcf-years).

Proportions of deaths attributable to mesotheliomas in cohort studies in the various mining and production sectors range from 0 to 0.8%. Caution should be exercised in interpreting these proportions, as studies do not provide comparable data stratifying deaths by exposure intensity, duration of exposure or time since first exposure.

There is evidence that fibrous tremolite causes mesothelioma in humans. Since commercial chrysotile may contain fibrous tremolite, it has been hypothesized that the latter may contribute to the induction of mesotheliomas in some populations exposed primarily to chrysotile. The extent to which the observed excesses of mesothelioma might be attributed to the fibrous tremolite content has not been resolved.

Epidemiological studies of populations of workers using chrysotile-containing products in applications such as construction have not been identified, although for workers with mixed exposures to chrysotile and the amphiboles, by far the greatest proportion of mesotheliomas occurs in users of asbestos-containing products rather than in those involved in their production.

9.3.2 General environment

Data on incidence or mortality of disease in household contacts of chrysotile workers or in populations exposed to airborne chrysotile in the vicinity of point sources reported since EHC 53 was published in 1986 have not been identified. More recent studies of populations exposed to chrysotile in drinking-water have likewise not been identified.

9.4 Effects on the environment

The impact of chrysotile/serpentine presence and degradation on the environment and lower life forms is difficult to gauge. Observed perturbations are many but their long-term impact is virtually unknown.

10. CONCLUSIONS AND RECOMMENDATIONS FOR PROTECTION OF HUMAN HEALTH

a) Exposure to chrysotile asbestos poses increased risks for asbestosis, lung cancer and mesothelioma in a dose-dependent manner. No threshold has been identified for carcinogenic risks.

b) Where safer substitute materials for chrysotile are available, they should be considered for use.

c) Some asbestos-containing products pose particular concern and chrysotile use in these circumstances is not recommended. These uses include friable products with high exposure potential. Construction materials are of particular concern for several reasons. The construction industry workforce is large and measures to control asbestos are difficult to institute. In-place building materials may also pose risk to those carrying out alterations, maintenance and demolition. Minerals in place have the potential to deteriorate and create exposures.

d) Control measures, including engineering controls and work practices, should be used in circumstances where occupational exposure to chrysotile can occur. Data from industries where control technologies have been applied have demonstrated the feasibility of controlling exposure to levels generally below 0.5 fibres/ml. Personal protective equipment can further reduce individual exposure where engineering controls and work practices prove insufficient.

e) Asbestos exposure and cigarette smoking have been shown to interact to increase greatly the risk of lung cancer. Those who have been exposed to asbestos can substantially reduce their lung cancer risk by avoiding smoking.

11. FURTHER RESEARCH

(a) Research and guidance are needed concerning the economic and practical feasibility of substitution for chrysotile asbestos, as well as the use of engineering controls and work practices in developing countries for controlling asbestos exposure.

(b) Further research is needed to understand more fully the molecular and cellular mechanisms by which asbestos causes fibrosis and cancer. The significance of physical and chemical properties (e.g., fibre dimension, surface properties) of fibres and their biopersistence in the lung to their biological and pathogenic effects needs further elucidation. Dose–response information from animal studies for various asbestos fibre types is needed to evaluate the differential risk of exposure to chrysotile and tremolite.

(c) Epidemiological studies of populations exposed to pure chrysotile (i.e. without appreciable amphiboles) are needed.

(d) The combined effects of chrysotile and other insoluble respirable particles needs further study.

(e) More epidemiological data are needed concerning cancer risks for populations exposed to fibre levels below 1 fibre/ml, as well as continued surveillance of asbestos-exposed populations.

REFERENCES

Abraham JL, Smith CM, & Mossman B (1988) Chrysotile and crocidolite asbestos pulmonary fibre concentrations and dimensions after inhalation and clearance in Fischer 344 rats. Ann Occup Hyg, **32** (suppl.1): 203-211.

Acheson ED, Gardner MJ, Pippard EC, & Grime LP (1982) Mortality of two groups of women who manufactured gas masks from chrysotile and crocidolite asbestos: a 40-year follow-up. Br J Ind Med, **39**: 344-348.

Adachi S, Kawamura K, Yoshida S, & Takemoto K (1992) Oxidative damage on DNA induced by asbestos and man-made fibres *in vitro*. Int Arch Occup Environ Health, **63**: 553-557.

Addison J & Davies ST (1990) Analysis of amphibole asbestos in chrysotile and other minerals. Ann Occup Hyg, **34**: 159-175.

AIA (1984) Method for the determination of airborne asbestos fibres and other inorganic fibres by scanning electron microscopy. London, Asbestos International Association, p 16.

AIA (1988) Reference method for the determination of airborne asbestos fibres concentrations at workplaces by light microscopy (membrane filter method). London, Asbestos International Association.

AIA (1995) AIA Proceedings of the 9th Biennial Conference. Montreal, 29-31 May 1995.

Albin M, Jakobsson K, Attewell R, Johansson L, & Wilinder H (1990) Mortality and cancer morbidity in cohorts of asbestos cement workers and referents. Br J Ind Med, **47**: 602-610.

Aliès-Patin AM & Valleron AJ (1985) Mortality of workers in a French asbestos cement factory 1940-1982. Br J Ind Med, **42**: 219-225.

Asgharian B & Yu CP (1988) Deposition of fibres in the rat lung. J Aerosol Med, **1**: 37-50.

Atkinson RJ (1973) Chrysotile asbestos: colloidal silica surfaces in acidified suspensions. J Colloid Interface Sci, **42**: 624-628.

Ayer HE, Lynch JR, & Fanney JH (1965) A comparison of impinger and membrane filter techniques for evaluating air samples in asbestos plants. Ann NY Acad Sci, **132**: 274-287.

Babich H & Stotzky G (1983) Toxicity of nickel to microbe: Environmental aspects. Adv Appl Microbiol, **29**: 195-266.

Bacon DW, Coomes OT, Marsan AA, & Rowlands N (1986) Assessing potential sources of asbestos fibers in water supplies of S.E. Quebec. Water Res Bull, **22**: 29-38.

Badollet MS (1948) Research on asbestos fibers. Can Min Metal Trans, **51**: 48-51.

Badollet MS & Gannt WA (1965) Preparation of asbestos fibres for experimental use. Ann Acad Sci, **132**: 451-455.

Bales RC & Morgan JJ (1985) Surface charge and adsorption properties of chrysotile asbestos in natural water. Environ Sci Technol, **19**: 1213-1219.

References

Baloyi R (1989) Exposure to asbestos among chrysotile miners, millers and mine residents and asbestosis in Zimbabwe. Helsinki, Institute of Occupational Health, University of Kuopio, pp 1-95 (Dissertation).

Becklake MR, Liddell FDK, Manfreda J, & McDonald JC (1979) Radiological changes after withdrawal from asbestos exposure. Br J Ind Med, 36: 23-28.

Becklake MR, Gibbs GW, Arhiri M, & Hurwitz S (1980) Respiratory changes in relation to asbestos exposure in manufacturing processes. Am Rev Respir Dis, 121: 223.

Begin R, Masse S, Rola-Pleszczynski M, Boctor M, & Drapeau G (1987) Asbestos exposure dose - bronchoalveolar milieu response in asbestos workers and the sheep model: evidences of a threshold for chrysotile-induced fibrosis. In: Fisher GL & Gallo MA ed. Asbestos toxicity. New York, Basel, Marcel Dekker Inc., pp 87-107.

Begin R, Masse S, Rola-Pleszczynski M, Drapeau G, & Dalle D (1985) Selective exposure and analysis of the sheep tracheal lobe as a model for toxicological studies of respirable particles. Environ Res, 36: 389-404.

Begin R, Masse S, Sebastien P, Bosse J, Rola-Pleszczynski M, Boctor M, Cote Y, Fabi D, & Dalle D (1986) Asbestos exposure and retention as determinants of airway disease and asbestos alveolitis. Am Rev Respir Dis, 134: 1176-1181.

Begin R, Cantin A, & Sebastien P (1990) Chrysotile asbestos exposures can produce an alveolitis with limited fibrosing activity in a subset of high fibre retainer sheep. Eur Respir J, 3: 81-90.

Begin R, Cantin A, & Masse S (1991) Influence of continued asbestos exposure on the outcome of asbestosis in sheep. Exp Lung Res, 17: 971-984.

Begin R, Gauthier JJ, Desmeules M, & Ostiguy G (1992) Work-related mesothelioma in Quebec 1967-90. Am J Ind Med, 22: 531-542.

Belanger SE, Cherry DS, & Cairns J (1986a) Uptake of chrysotile asbestos fibers alters growth and reproduction of Asiatic clams. Can J Fish Aquat Sci, 43: 43-52.

Belanger SE, Cherry DS, & Cairns J (1986b) Seasonal, behavioral and growth changes of juvenile Corbicula fluminea exposed to chrysotile asbestos. Water Res, 20: 1243-1250.

Belanger SE, Schurr K, Allen DJ, & Gohara AF (1986c) Effects of chrysotile asbestos on Coho salmon and green sunfish: evidence of behavioral and pathological stress. Environ Res, 39: 74-83.

Belanger SE, Cherry DS, Cairns J, & McGuire MJ (1987) Using Asiatic clams as a biomonitor for chrysotile asbestos in public water supplies. J Am Water Works Assoc, 79: 69-74.

Belanger SE, Cherry DS, & Cairns J Jr (1990) Functional and pathological impairment of Japanese Medaka (Oryzias latipes) by long-term asbestos exposure. Aquat Toxicol, 17: 133-154.

Bellmann B, Muhle H, Pott F, Konig H, Kloppel H, & Sourny K (1987) Persistence of man-made mineral fibres and asbestos in rat lungs. Ann Occup Hyg, 31: 693-709.

Berry G & Newhouse ML (1983) Mortality of workers manufacturing friction products using asbestos. Br J Ind Med, 40: 1-7.

Berry G, Gilson JC, Holmes S, Lewinsohn HC, & Roach SA (1979) Asbestosis: a study of dose-response relationships in an asbestos textile factory. Br J Ind Med, 36: 98-112.

Berry G, Newhouse M, & Antonis P (1985) Combined effects of asbestos and smoking on mortality from lung cancer and mesothelioma in factory workers. Br J Ind Med, 42: 12-18.

Bérubé KA, Quinlan TR, Mouton G, Hemenway D, o'Shaughnessy P, Vacek P, & Mossman BT (1996) Comparative proliferative and histopathologic changes in rat lungs after inhalation of chrysotile or crocidolite asbestos. Oncol Appl Pharmacol, 137: 67-74.

Bignon J & Brochard P (1995) Enquête cas-témoins multicentrique portant sur le mésothéliome pleural: période 1987-1993. Report to the French Ministry of Health.

Bignon J, Monchaux G, Hirsch A, Sebastien P, & Lafuma J (1979) Human and experimental data on translocation of asbestos fibres through the respiratory system. Ann NY Acad Sci, 330: 745-770.

Bissonnette E, Dubois C, & Rola-Pleszczynski M (1989) Changes in lymphocyte function and lung histology during the development of asbestosis and silicosis in the mouse. Res Commun Chem Pathol Pharmacol, 65: 211-227.

Boatman ES, Merril T, O'Neill A, Polissar L, & Millette JR (1983) Use of quantitative analysis of urine to assess exposure to asbestos fibers in drinking water in the Puget Sound region. Environ Health Pespect, 53: 131-139.

Bohning DE, Atkins HL, & Cohn SH (1982) Long-term particle clearance in man: normal and impaired. Ann Occup Hyg, 26: 259-271.

Bolton RE, Davis JM, & Lamb D (1982) The pathological effects of prolonged asbestos ingestion in rats. Environ Res, 29: 134-150.

Bonner JC & Brody AR (1991) Asbestos-induced alveolar injury - evidence from macrophage-derived PDGF as a mediator of the fibrogenic response. Chest, 99: 54-55.

Bonner JC, Goodell AL, Coin PG, & Brody AR (1993) Chrysotile asbestos up-regulates gene expression and production of alpha-receptors for platelet-derived growth factor (pdgf-aa) on rat lung fibroblasts. J Clin Invest, 92: 425-430.

Bordeleau LM, LaLande R, DeKimpe CR, Zizka J, & Tabi M (1977) Effets des poussières d'amiante sur la microflore tellurique. Plant Soil, 46: 619-627.

Boutin C, Dumortier P, Rey F, Viallat JR, & De Vuyst P (1993) Oncogenic asbestos fibers in the parietal pleura. In: Proceedings of a Workshop on Cellular and Molecular Effects of Minerals and Synthetic Dusts and Fibres. Paris, Moncassin.

Bowes DR, Langer AM, & Rohl AN (1977) Nature and range of mineral dusts in the environment. Philos Trans R Soc (Lond), A286: 593-610.

Bozelka BE, Sestini P, Hammad Y, & Salvaggio JE (1986) Effects of asbestos fibers on alveolar macrophage-mediated lymphocyte cytostasis. Environ Res, 40: 172-180.

Bravo M, Del Rey-Calero J, & Conde M (1988) Bladder cancer and asbestosis in Spain. Rev Epidémiol Santé Publique, 36: 10-14.

References

Brody AR & Overby LH (1989) Incorporation of tritiated thymidine by epithelial and interstitial cells in bronchiolar-alveolar regions of asbestos exposed rats. Am J Pathol, **134**: 133-140.

Brody AR & Roe MW (1983) Deposition pattern of inorganic particles at the alveolar level in the lungs of rats and mice. Am Rev Respir Dis, **128**: 724-729.

Brody AR, Hill LH, Adkins B Jr, & O'Connor RW (1981) Chrysotile asbestos inhalation in rats: deposition pattern and reaction of alveolar epithelium and pulmonary macrophages. Am Rev Respir Dis, **123**: 670-679.

Brooks RR (1987) Serpentine and its vegetation. Portland, Oregon, Dioscorides Press Ltd, 454 pp.

Brown LM, Dement J, & Okun A (1994) Mortality patterns among female and male asbestos textile workers. J Occup Med, **36**: 882-888.

Bunn WB, Bender JR, Hesterberg TW, Chase GR, & Konzen JL (1993) Recent studies of man-made vitreous fibers: Chronic animals inhalation studies. J Occup Med, **35**: 101-113.

Burdett GJ & Jaffrey SAMT (1986) Airborne asbestos concentrations in public buildings. Ann Occup Hyg, **30**: 185-190.

Burger BF & Engelbrecht FM (1970) The biological effects of long and short fibres of crocidolite and chrysotile A after intrapleural injection into rats. S Afr Med J, **44**: 1268-1278.

Canada Environmental Health Directorate (1979) A national survey for asbestos fibres in Canadian drinking-water. Ottawa, Canada, Environmental Health Directorate.

Cantin A, Dubois F, & Begin R (1988) Lung exposure to mineral dusts enhances the capacity of lung inflammatory cells to release superoxide. J Leukoc Biol, **43**: 299-303.

Cantin A, Allard C, & Begin R (1989) Increased alveolar plasminogen activator in early asbestosis. Am Rev Respir Dis, **139**: 604-609.

Case BW, Kuhar M, Harrigan M, & Defresne A (1994) Lung fibre content of American children aged 8-15: preliminary findings. In: Dodgson J & McCallum RI ed. Proceedings of the 7th BOHS Inhaled Particles Symposium, Edinburgh. Ann Occup Hyg, **38**(4): 639-645.

CEC (1983) Council directive on the protection of workers from the risks related to exposure to asbestos at work. Off J Eur Communities, **L263**: 25.

Chang LY, Overby LH, Brody AR, & Crapo JD (1988) Progressive lung cell reactions and extracellular matrix production after a brief exposure to asbestos. Am J Pathol, **131**: 156-169.

Chatfield E (1979) Measurement of asbestos fibres in the workplace and in the general environment. In: Ledoux RL ed. Short course in mineralogical techniques of asbestos determination. Ottawa, Mineralogical Association of Canada, pp 111-163.

Chatfield E (1986) Airborne asbestos levels in Canadian public buildings. In: Chatfield E ed. Asbestos fibres measurements in building atmospheres - Proceedings. Mississauga, Ontario, Ontario Research Foundation, pp 177-207.

Chatfield E (1987) Limits of detection and precision in monitoring for asbestos fibers. In: Asbestosis - its health risks, analysis, regulation and control. Proceeding of APCA Specialty Conference. Atlantic City, New York, Air Pollution Control Association, pp 79-90.

Chen L, Li Q, Hu T, & Guo J (1988) [A historical prospective investigation of malignant tumours in a Shanghai asbestos product factory.] Labour Med, **1**: 6-9 (in Chinese).

Cheng W & Kong J (1992) A retrospective mortality cohort study of chrysotile asbestos products workers in Tianjin 1972-1987. Environ Res, **59**: 271-278.

Cheng VKI & O'Kelly FJ (1986) Asbestos exposure in the motor vehicle repair and servicing industry in Hong Kong. J Soc Occup Med, **36**: 104-106.

Chesson J, Margeson DP, Ogden J, Bauer K, Constant PC, Bergman FJ, & Rose DP (1985) Evaluation of asbestos abatement techniques. Phase 1: Removal. Washington, DC, US Environmental Protection Agency (EPA-560/5-85-109).

Chesson J, Hatfield J, Schultz B, Dutrow E, & Blake J (1990) Airborne asbestos in public buildings. Environ Res, **51**: 100-107.

Chiappino G, Todaro A, & Sebastien P (1993) The levels of asbestos fibres in Italian towns: what is the level of risk? In: Gibbs WH, Dunnigan J, Kido M, & Higashi T ed. Health risks from exposure to mineral fibres. North York, Captus Press Inc., pp 120-128.

Churchyard MP & Copeland GKE (1988) Is it really chrysotile? Ann Occup Hyg, **32**: 545-547

Churg A (1994) Deposition and clearance of chrysotile asbestos. Ann Occup Hyg, **38**: 625-633.

Churg A & DePaoli L (1988) Clearance of chrysotile asbestos from human lung. Exp Lung Res, **14**: 567-574.

Churg A, Wright JL, Gilks B, & DePaoli L (1989) Rapid short term clearance of chrysotile compared to amosite asbestos in the guinea pig. Am Rev Respir Dis, **139**: 885-890.

Churg A, Wright JL, & Vedal S (1993) Fiber burden and patterns of asbestos-related disease in chrysotile miners and millers. Am Rev Respir Dis, **148**: 25-31.

Clemmensen J & Hjalgrim-Jensen S (1981) Cancer incidence among 5686 asbestos-cement workers followed from 1943 through 1976. Ecotoxicol Environ Saf, **5**: 15-23.

Coffin DL, Cook PM, & Creason JP (1992) Relative mesothelioma induction in rats by mineral fibres: comparison with residual pulmonary mineral fibre number and epidemiology. Inhal Toxicol, **4**: 273-300.

Cohen D, Arai S, & Brain JD (1979) Smoking impairs long-term dust clearance from the lung. Science, **204**: 97-116.

Coin PG, Roggli VL, & Brody AR (1992) Deposition, clearance and translocation of chrysotile asbestos from peripheral and central regions of the rat lung. Environ Res, **58**: 97-116.

Coin PG, Roggli VL, & Brody AR (1994) Persistence of long thin chrysotile asbestos fibres in the lungs of rats. Environ Health Perspect, **102**(Suppl 5): 197-199.

Commins BT & Gibbs GW (1969) Contaminating organic material in asbestos. Br J Cancer, **23**: 358-362.

Condie LW (1983) Review of published studies of orally administered asbestos. Environ Health Perspect, **53**: 3-9.

Cook PM (1983) Review of published studies on gut penetration by ingested asbestos fibres. Environ Health Perspect, **53**: 121-130.

Cooper TC, Sheehy JW, O'Brien DM, McGlothlin JD, & Todd WF (1988) In-depth survey report: evaluation of brake drum service controls at Cincinnati gas and electric garages. Cincinnati, Ohio, National Institute of Occupational Safety and Health (Report CT-152-22b).

Cordier S, Theriault G, & Provencher S (1984) Radiographic changes in a group of chrysotile miners and millers exposed to low asbestos concentrations. Br J Ind Med, **41**: 384-388.

Corn M (1994) Airborne concentrations of asbestos in nonoccupational environments. Ann Occup Hyg, **38**: 495-502.

Corn M, Crump K, Farrar DB, Lee RJ, & McFee DR (1991) Airborne concentrations of asbestos in 71 school buildings. Regul Toxicol Pharmacol, **13**: 99-114.

Corn M, McArthur B, & Dellarco M (1994) Asbestos exposures in building maintenance personnel. Appl Occup Environ Hyg, **9**: 845-852.

Corpet DE, Perot V, & Goubet I (1993) Asbestos induces aberrant crypt foci in the colon of rats. Cancer Lett, **74(3)**: 183-187.

Cossette M & Delvaux P (1979) Technical evaluation of chrysotile asbestos ore bodies. In: Ledoux RL ed. Short course in mineralogical techniques of asbestos determination. Ottawa, Mineralogical Association of Canada, pp 79-110.

Cossette M, Delvaux P, VanHa T, L'Esperance C, & Belleville GG (1986) Physiological innocuity of asbestos in water. Nordeast Environ Sci, **5**: 54-62.

Cralley LJ, Keenan RG, & Lynch JR (1967) Exposure to metals and the manufacture of asbestos textile products. Am Ind Hyg Assoc J, **28**: 452-461.

Crump KS & Farrar DB (1989) Statistical analysis of data on airborne asbestos levels collected in an EPA survey of public buildings. Regul Toxicol Pharmacol, **10**: 51-62.

CPSC (1987) Report on the first round of air sampling of asbestos in home study. Washington, DC, US Consumer Product Safety Commission.

Cullen MR & Baloyi R (1991) Chrysotile asbestos and health in Zimbabwe: I. Analysis of miners and millers compensated for asbestos-related diseases since independence (1980). Am J Ind Med, **19**: 161-169.

Cullen MR, Lopez-Carillo L, Alli B, Pace PE, Shlat SL, & Baloyi RS (1991) Chrysotile asbestos and health in Zimbabwe: II. Health status survey of active miners and millers. Am J Ind Med, **19**: 171-182.

Dagbert M (1976) Etudes de corrélation de mesures d'empoussiérage dans l'industrie de l'amiante. Montréal, Comité d'Etude sur la Salubrité dans l'Industrie de l'Amiante, 114 pp. (Document 5).

Davis JMG (1972) The fibrogenic effects of mineral dust injected into the pleural cavity of mice. Br J Exp Pathol, **53**: 190-195.

Davis JMG (1989) Mineral fibres carcinogenesis: Experimental data relating to the importance of fibre type, size, deposition, dissolution and migration. In: Bignon J, Peto J, & Saracci R ed. Non-occupational exposure to mineral fibres. Lyon, International Agency for Research on Cancer, pp 33-45 (IARC Scientific Publications No. 90).

Davis JMG (1993) Information from experimental studies relating to the effects of ingestion of mineral fibres. In: Gibbs GW, Dunnigan J, Kido M, & Higashi T ed. Health risks from exposure to mineral fibres - an International Perspective. North York, Captus University Publications, pp 152-163.

Davis JMG & Cowie H (1990) The relationship between fibrosis and cancer in experimental animals exposed to asbestos and other fibers. Environ Health Perspect, **88**: 305-309.

Davis JMG & Jones AD (1988) Comparisons of the pathogenicity of long and short fibre of chrysotile asbestos in rats. Br J Exp Pathol, **69**: 717-737.

Davis JMG, Beckett ST, Bolton RE, Collings P, & Middleton AP (1978) Mass and number of fibres in the pathogenesis of asbestos-related lung disease in rats. Br J Cancer, **37**: 673-688.

Davis JMG, Beckett ST, Bolton RE, & Donaldson K (1980) The effects of intermittent high asbestos exposure (peak dose levels) on the lungs of rats. Br J Exp Pathol, **61**: 272-280.

Davis JMG, Addison J, Bolton RE, Donaldson K, Jones AD, & Miller BG (1985) Inhalation studies on the effects of tremolite and brucite dust in rats. Carcinogenesis, **5**: 667-674.

Davis JMG, Addison J, Bolton RE, Donaldson K, & Jones AD (1986a) Inhalation and injection studies in rats using dust samples from chrysotile asbestos prepared by a wet dispersion process. Br J Exp Pathol, **67**: 113-129.

Davis JMG, Addison J, Bolton RE, Donaldson K, Jones AD, & Smith T (1986b) The pathogenicity of long versus short fibre samples of amosite asbestos administered to rats by inhalation and intraperitoneal injection. Br J Exp Pathol, **67**: 473-491.

Davis JMG, Bolton RE, Douglas AN, Jones AD, & Smith T (1988) The effects of electrostatic charge on the pathogenicity of chrysotile asbestos. Br J Ind Med, **45**: 337-345.

Davis JMG, Bolton RE, Brown DM, Brown GM, Donaldson K, Jones AD, Robertson MD, & Slight J (1989) *In vitro* studies of leucocytes lavaged from the lungs of rats following the inhalation of mineral dusts. In: Mossman BT & Begin RO ed. Effects of mineral dusts on cells. Berlin, Heildelberg, New York, Springer-Verlag, pp 337-345.

Davis JMG, Jones AD, & Miller BG (1991a) Experimental studies in rats on the effects of asbestos inhalation coupled with the inhalation of titanium dioxide or quartz. Int J Exp Pathol, **72**: 501-525.

Davis JMG, Bolton RE, Miller BG, & Niven K (1991b) Mesothelioma dose response following intraperitoneal injection of mineral fibres. Int J Exp Pathol, **72**: 263-274.

References

Davis JMG, Addison J, McIntosh C, Miller BGM, & Niven K (1991c) Variations in the carcinogenicity of tremolite dust samples of different morphology. Ann NY Acad Sci, 37: 673-689.

Day R, Lemaire I, Masse S, & Lemaire S (1985) Pulmonary bombesin in experimentally induced asbestosis in rats. Exp Lung Res, 8: 1-13.

Day R, Lemaire S, Nadeau D, Keith I, & Lemaire I (1987) Changes in autacoid and neuropeptide contents of lung cells in asbestos-induced pulmonary fibrosis. Am Rev Respir Dis, 136: 908-915.

Dement JM (1991) Carcinogenicity of chrysotile asbestos: a case-control study of textile workers. Cell Biol Toxicol, 7: 59-65.

Dement JM & Wallingford KM (1990) Comparison of phase contrast and electron microscopic methods for evaluation of occupational asbestos exposures. Appl Occup Environ Hyg, 5(4): 242-247.

Dement JM, Harris RL, Symons MJ, & Shy CM (1983a) Exposures and mortality among chrysotile asbestos workers. Part I: Exposure estimates. Am J Ind Med, 4: 399-419.

Dement JM, Harris RL, Symons MJ, & Shy CM (1983b) Exposures and mortality among chrysotile asbestos workers. Part II: Mortality. Am J Ind Med, 4: 421-433.

Dement JM, Brown DP, & Okun A (1994) Follow-up study of chrysotile asbestos textile workers: cohort mortality and case-control analyses. Am J Ind Med, 26: 431-447.

Deom E (1989) Plant diversity and mycorrhizal status of serpentine and adjacent soils. University of British Columbia, Department of Soil Science, 75 pp (BSc Thesis).

Dodson RF, Williams MG, Corn CJ, Brollo A, & Bianchi C (1990) Asbestos content of lung tissue, lymph nodes, and pleural plaques from former shipyard workers. Am Rev Respir Dis, 142: 843-847.

Doll R (1955) Mortality from lung cancer in asbestos workers. Br J Ind Med, 12: 81-86.

Doll R & Peto J (1985) Effects on health of exposure to asbestos. London, Her Majesty's Stationery Office, Health & Safety Commission, pp 1-58.

Donaldson K, Bolton RE, Jones A, Brown GM, Robertson MD, Slight J, Cowie H, & Davis JMG (1988a) Kinetics of the bronchoalveolar leucocyte response in rats during exposure to equal airborne mass concentrations of quartz, chrysotile asbestos or titanium dioxide. Thorax, 43: 525-533.

Donaldson K, Slight J, Brown GM, & Bolton RE (1988b) The ability of inflammatory bronchoalveolar leucocyte populations elicited with microbes or mineral dust to injure alveolar epithelial cells and degrade extracellular matrix *in vitro*. Br J Exp Pathol, 69: 327-338.

Donaldson K, Brown GM, Brown DM, Slight J, Robertson MD, & Davis IMG (1990) Impaired chemotactic responses of bronchoalveolar leukocytes in experimental pneumoconiosis. J Pathol, 160: 63-69.

Donham KJ, Berg JW, Will LA, & Leininger JR (1980) The effects of long-term ingestion of asbestos on the colon of F344 rats. Cancer, 45: 1073.

Dreesen WC, Dalavalle JW, Edwards TI, Miller JW, & Sayers RR (1938) A study of asbestos in the asbestos textile industry. Washington, DC, US Public Health Service (Public Health Bulletin No. 241).

Dubois CM, Bissonnette E, & Rola-Pleszczynski P (1989) Asbestos fibers and silica particles stimulate rat alveolar macrophages to release tumor necrosis factor. Am Rev Respir Dis, **139**: 1257-1264.

Du Toit RSJ & Gilfillan TC (1979) Conversion of asbestos fibre concentrations recorded by means of the konimeter and the thermal precipitator to that expected by means of the membrane filter method. Ann Occup Hyg, **22**: 67-83.

Du Toit RSJ, Isserow LW, Gilfillan TC, Robock K, & Teichert U (1983) Relationships between simultaneous airborne dust sample taken with 5 types of instruments at South African asbestos mines and mills. Ann Occup Hyg, **27**: 373-387.

Elliehausen HJ, Paur R, Roedelsperger K, & Woitowitz HJ (1985) [The risk of sequelae of asbestos inhalation in motor mechanics working in brake services.] Arb. med Soz. med Praev. med, **20**: 256-261 (in German).

Enarson DA, Embree V, Maclean L, & Grzybowski S (1988) Respiratory health in chrysotile asbestos miners in British Columbia: a longitudinal study. Br J Ind Med, **45**: 459-463.

Enterline PE, Hartley J, & Henderson V (1987) Asbestos and cancer: A cohort followed up to death. Br J Ind Med, **44**: 396-401.

Fasske E (1988) Experimental lung tumors following specific intrabronchial application of chrysotile asbestos. Respiration, **53**: 111-127.

Fatma N, Khan SG, Aslam M, & Rahman Q (1992) Induction of chromosomal aberrations in bone marrow cells of asbestotic rats. Environ Res, **57**: 175-180.

Fei H & Huang JQ (1989) [A study on the relationship between gravimetric and fibre concentrations of airborne dust in asbestos paper industry.] Gongye Weisheng Yu Zhiyebing, **15**(6): 339-343 (in Chinese).

Finkelstein M (1983) Mortality among long-term employees of an Ontario asbestos-cement factory. Br J Ind Med, **40**: 138-144.

Finkelstein M (1984) Mortality among employees of an Ontario asbestos-cement factory. Am Rev Respir Dis, **129**: 754-761.

Finn MB & Hallenbeck WH (1985) Detection of chrysotile asbestos in workers' urine. Am Ind Hyg Assoc J, **46**(3): 162-169.

Frank AL (1995) The use of asbestos in Japan and China and malignancy related findings. Med Lav, **85**: 457-460.

Gardner MJ, Winter PD, Pannett B, & Powell CA (1986) Follow-up study of workers manufacturing chrysotile asbestos cement product. Br J Ind Med, **43**: 726-732.

Gasser U, Juchler SJ, Hobson WA, & Sticher H (1995) The fate of chromium and nickel in subalpine soils derived from serpentine. Can J Soil Sci, **75**: 187-195.

References

Gaudichet A, Sebastien P, Clark NJ, & Pooley FD (1980) Identification and quantification of asbestos in human tissues. In: Wagner JC ed. Biological effects of mineral fibres. Lyon, International Agency for Research on Cancer, vol 2, pp 61-88 (IARC Scientific Publications No 30).

Gazzi D & Crockford GW (1987) Indoor asbestos levels on a housing estate (determined by transmission electron microscopy). Ann Occup Hyg, **31**(4A): 429-439.

Gerde P & Scholander P (1989) A model for the influence of inhaled mineral fibers on the pulmonary uptake of polycyclic aromatic hydrocarbons (PAH) from cigarette smoke. In: Wehner AP & Felton DV ed. Biological interaction of inhaled fibers and cigarette smoke. Richland, Washington, Battelle Pacific, pp 97-120.

Gibbs GW (1971a) Qualitative aspects of dust exposure in the Quebec asbestos mining and milling industry. In: Walton WH ed. Inhaled particles III. Surrey, Unwin Brothers Ltd, pp 783-799.

Gibbs GW (1971b) The organic geochemistry of chrysotile asbestos from eastern townships, Quebec. Geochim Cosmochim Acta, **35**: 585-502.

Gibbs GW (1994) The assessment of exposure in terms of fibres. Ann Occup Hyg, **38**: 477-487.

Gibbs GW & Hui HY (1971) The organic content of Canadian chrysotile. Am Ind Hyg Assoc J, **32**: 519-528.

Gibbs GW & Hwang CY (1980) Dimensions of airborne asbestos fibres. In: Wagner JC ed. Biological effects of mineral fibres. Lyon, International Agency for Research on Cancer, pp 69-77 (IARC Scientific Publication No. 30).

Gibbs GW & Lachance M (1972) Dust exposure in the chrysotile asbestos mines and mills of Quebec. Arch Environ Health, **24**: 189-197.

Gibbs GW & Lachance M (1974) Dust-fibre relationships in Quebec chrysotile industry. Arch Environ Health, **28**: 69-71.

Godbey FW, Cooper TC, Sheehy JWE, O'Brien DM, Van Wagenen HD, McGlothlin JD, & Todd WF (1987) In-depth survey report: Evaluation of brake drum service controls at United States postal service vehicle maintenance facility Nashville. Cincinnati, Ohio, National Institute of Occupational Safety and Health (Report CT-152-20b).

Goldstein B & Coetzee FSJ (1990) Experimental malignant mesothelioma in baboons. Suid-Afr Tydskr Wet, **86**: 89-93.

Gorski CH & Stettler LE (1974) The adsorption of water and benzene on amosite and chrysotile asbestos. Am Ind Hyg Assoc J, **35**: 354-361.

Graney RJ, Cherry DS, & Crains J (1983) Heavy metal indicator potential of the Asiatic clam (*Corbicula fluminea*) in artificial stream systems. Hydrobiologia, **102**: 81-85.

Gulumian M & Van Wyk JA (1987) Hydroxyl radical production in the presence of fibres by a fenton-type reaction. Chem-Biol Interact, **62**: 89-97.

Hallenbeck WH, Chen EH, Patel-Mandlik K, & Wolff AH (1977) Precision of analysis for waterborne chrysotile asbestos by transmission electron microscopy. Bull Environ Contam Toxicol, 17: 551-558.

Hammad YY, Diem H, & Weill H (1979) Evaluation of dust exposure in asbestos cement manufacturing operations. Am Ind Hyg Assoc J, 40: 490-495.

Hannant D, Donaldson K, & Bolton RE (1985) Immunomodulatory effects of mineral dust. Effects of intraperitoneal dust inoculation on splenic lymphocyte function and humoral immune responses in vivo. J Clin Immunol, 16: 81-85.

Harrison PTC & Heath JC (1988) Apparent synergy between chrysotile asbestos and N-nitroheptamethyleneimine in the induction of pulmonary tumours in rats. Carcinogenesis, 9: 2165-2171.

Hartmann DP, Georgian MM, Oghiso Y, & Kagan E (1984a) Enhanced interleukin activity following asbestos inhalation. Clin Exp Immunol, 55: 643-650.

Hartmann DP, Georgian MM, & Kagan E (1984b) Enhanced alveolar macrophage Ia antigen expression after asbestos inhalation. J Immunol, 132: 2693-2695.

Harvey G, Page M, & Dumas L (1984) Binding of environmental carcinogens to asbestos and mineral fibres. Br J Ind Med, 41: 396-400.

Hatfield J, Ogden J, Srockrahm J, Leczynski B, Price B, Chesson J, Russel J, Ford P, Thomas J, Fitzgerald J, Roat R, Lee R, Van Orden D, Dunmyre G, Constant P, & McHugh J (1988) Assessing asbestos exposure in public buildings. Washington, DC, US Environmental Protection Agency (EPA-560/5-88-002).

Hays AA, Venaille TJ, Rose AH, Musk AW, & Robinson WS (1990) Asbestos-induced release of a human alveolar macrophage-derived neutrophil chemotactic factor. Exp Lung Res, 16: 121-130.

Hayward SB (1984) Field monitoring of chrysotile asbestos in California waters. J Am Water Work Assoc, 76: 66-73.

HEI (1991) Asbestos in public and commercial buildings: A literature review and synthesis of current knowledge. Cambridge, Massachusetts, Health Effects Institute-Asbestos Research.

Hei TK, Piao CQ, He ZY, Vannais D, & Waldren, C (1992) Chrysotile fiber is a strong mutagen in mammalian cells. Cancer Res, 52: 6305-6309.

Heintz NH, Janssen YM, & Mossman BT (1993) Persistent induction of c-fos and c-jun expression by asbestos. Proc Natl Acad Sci (USA), 90: 3299-3303.

Henderson DW, De Klerk NH, Hammar SP, Hillerdal G, Huuskonen MS, Leigh J, Pott F, Roggli VL, Shilkin KB, & Tossavainen A (1996) Asbestos and lung cancer: an old controversy revisited. In press.

Henderson DW, de Klerk NH, Hammar SP, Hillerdal G, Huuskonen MS, Leigh J, Pott F, Roggli VL, Shilkin KB, & Tossavainen A (1997) Asbestos and lung cancer: Is it attributable to asbestosis or to asbestos fiber burden? In: Corrin B ed. Pathology of lung tumors. New York, Edinburgh, London, Churchill Livingstone, pp 83-118.

References

Herman RL (1985) Mesothelioma in rainbow trout, *Salmo gairdneri* Richardson. J Fish Dis, 8(4): 373-376.

Hesse CS, Hallenbeck WH, Chen EH, & Brenniman GR (1977) Determination of chrysotile asbestos in rain water. Atmos Environ, 11: 1233-1237.

Hesterberg TW, Mast R, McConnell EE, Chevalier J, Bernstein DM, Bunn WB, & Anderson R (1991) Chronic inhalation toxicity of refractory ceramic fibers in Syrian hamsters. In: Brown RC, Hoskin JA, & Johnson NF ed. Mechanisms of fibre carcinogenesis. New York, Plenum Press, pp 531-539.

Hesterberg TW, Miller WC, McConnell EE, Chevalier J, Hadley JG, Bernstein DM, Thevenaz P, & Anderson R (1993) Chronic inhalation toxicity of size-separated glass fibers in Fischer 344 rats. Fundam Appl Toxicol, 20: 464-476.

Higashi T, Hori H, Sakurai H, Omae K, Tsuda T, Tanaka T, Tanaka I, Satoh T, & Hoshi H (1994) Work environment of plants manufacturing asbestos-containing products in Japan. Ann Occup Hyg, 38: 489-494.

Hirano S, Ono M, & Aimoto A (1988) Functional and biochemical effects on rat lungs following instillation of crocidolite and chrysotile asbestos. J Toxicol Environ Health, 24: 27-39.

Hiroshima KK, Murai Y, Suzuki Y, Goldstein B, & Webster I (1993) Characterization of asbestos fibers in lungs and mesotheliomatous tissues of baboons following long-term inhalation. Am J Ind Med, 23: 883-901.

HSE (Health and Safety Executive) (1979) Asbestos - Volume 1: Final report of the Advisory Committee. London, Her Majesty's Stationary Office.

Huang JQ (1990) A study on the dose-response relationship between asbestos exposure level and asbestosis among workers in a Chinese chrysotile product factory. Biomed Environ Sci, 3: 90-98.

Hughes JM & Weill H (1991) Asbestosis as a precursor of asbestos related lung cancer: Results of a prospective mortality study. Br J Ind Med, 48: 229-233.

Hughes JM, Weill H, & Hammad YY (1987) Mortality of workers employed in two asbestos cement manufacturing plants. Br J Ind Med, 44: 161-174.

Huilan Z & Zhiming W (1993) Study of occupational lung cancer in asbestos factories in China. Br J Ind Med, 50: 1039-1042.

Hume LA & Rimstidt JD (1992) The biodurability of chrysotile asbestos. Am Miner, 77: 1125-1128.

IARC (1996) In: Kane AB, Saracci R, Boffetta P, & Wilbourn JD ed. Mechanisms of fibre carcinogenesis. Lyon, International Agency for Research on Cancer (IARC Publication No. 40).

ILO (1984) Safety in the use of asbestos. Geneva, International Labour Office, 120 pp.

Industrial Minerals (1990) Asbestos cement markets, full of Eastern promise.

Industrial Minerals (1992) Asbestos production: the chrysotile crisis?

IPCS (1986) Environmental health criteria 53: Asbestos and other natural mineral fibres. Geneva, World Health Organization, International Programme on Chemical Safety, 194 pp.

IPCS (1988) Environmental health criteria 77: Man-made mineral fibres. Geneva, World Health Organization, International Programme on Chemical Safety, 165 pp.

IPCS (1989) Reduction of asbestos in the environment. Geneva, World Health Organization, International Programme on Chemical Safety, 151 pp (ICS/89.34).

IPCS (1993) Environmental health criteria 151: Selected synthetic organic fibres. Geneva, World Health Organization, International Programme on Chemical Safety, 100 pp.

ISO (1991) Ambient air - Determination of asbestos fibres: direct transfer transmission electron microscopy procedure. Geneva, International Standard Organization, 85 pp (ISO/DP10312).

ISO (1992) Ambient air: measurement of inorganic fibrous particles - scanning electron microscopy method. Geneva, International Standard Organization, 50 pp (ISO/TC I46 SC 3/WG1-N35).

ISO (1993) Workplace atmospheres, determination of asbestos, phase contrast procedure. Geneva, International Standard Organization, 20 pp (ISO/TC 146/SC 2).

Jacobs R, Humphrys S, Dogson KS, & Richards RJ (1978) Light and electron microscope studies of the rat digestive tract following prolonged and short-term ingestion of chrysotile asbestos. Br J Exp Pathol, **59**: 443-453.

Jakobsson K, Albin M, & Hagmar L (1994) Asbestos, cement, and cancer in the right part of the colon. J Environ Med, **51**: 95-101.

Jaffrey SAMT (1988) Releasibility of asbestos fiber - Occupational medicine and hygiene laboratory. London, UK Health and Safety Executive (IR/L/DI/88/12).

Jaffrey SAMT (1990) Environmental asbestos fiber release from brake and clutch linings of vehicular traffic. Ann Occup Hyg, **34**: 529-534.

Jahn H, Roedelsperger K, Bruckel B, Manke J, & Woitowitz HJ (1985) [Asbestos dust risks in brake repair services.] Staub-Reinhalt Luft, **45**: 80-83 (in German).

Jaurand MC, Bignon J, Sebastien P, & Goni J (1977) Leaching of chrysotile asbestos in human lungs: correlation with in vitro studies using rabbit alveolar macrophages. Environ Res, **14**: 245-254.

Jaurand MC, Kheuang L, Magne L, & Bignon J (1986) Chromosomal changes induced by chrysotile fibres or benzo(3-4)pyrene in rat pleural mesothelial cells. Mutat Res, **169**: 141-145.

Jaurand MC, Yegles M, & Dong HY (1994) In vitro DNA and chromosome damage produced by some minerals and man-made particles on rat pleural mesothelial cells (RPMC): Mechanism and relationship with in vivo experimental findings. In: Davis JMG & Jaurand MC ed. Cellular and molecular effects of mineral and synthetic dusts and fibres. Berlin, Heidelberg, Springer-Verlag, pp 183-192 (NATO ASI Series, Volume H85).

Jones J & McGuire MJ (1987) Dredging to reduce asbestos concentrations in the Californian aqueduct. J Am Water Work Assoc, **79**: 30-37.

Jones AD, Johnston AM, & Vincent JH (1983) Static electrification of airborne asbestos dust. In: Marple VA & Liu BYH ed. Aerosols in the mining and industrial work environment. Ann Arbor, Michigan, Ann Arbor Science Publishers Inc., vol 2, pp 613-632.

Jones RN, Diem JE, Hughes JM, Hammad YY, Glindmeyer HW, & Weill H (1989) Progression of asbestos effects: A prospective longitudinal study of chest radiographs and lung function. Br J Ind Med, **46**: 97-105.

Jones AD, Vincent JH, Addison J, McIntosh C, & Donaldson K (1994) The fate and effect of inhaled chrysotile asbestos fibres. Ann Occup Hyg, **38**(suppl 1): 619-629.

Juck A, Cambelova M, & Ulrich L (1991) Practice of determination and evaluation of asbestos and MMMF in the Slovak Republic. In: Proceedings of the AIA/NIOH International Colloquium on Dust Measurement Techniques and Strategy. Budapest, National Institute of Occupational Health, pp 83-94.

Julian Y & McCrone WC (1970) Identification of asbestos fibres by microscopical dispersion staining. Microscope, **18**: 1-11.

Kaplan H, Renier A, Jaurand MC, & Bignon J (1980) Sister chromatid exchanges in mesothelial cells cultured with chrysotile asbestos. In: Brown RC, Gormeley IP, Chamberlain M, & Daviers R ed. The *in vitro* effects of mineral dusts. New York, London, Academic Press, pp 152-253.

Kasai H & Nishimura S (1984) DNA damage induced by asbestos in the presence of hydrogen peroxide. Gann, **75**: 841-844.

Kauffer E, Vigneron JC, Hesbert A, & Lemorimer M (1987) A study of the length and diameter of fibres in lung and in bronchoalveolar lavage fluid, following exposure of rats to chrysotile asbestos. Ann Occup Hyg, **31**: 233-240.

Kauppinen T & Korhonen K (1987) Exposure to asbestos during brake maintenance of automotive vehicles by different methods. Am Ind Hyg Assoc J, **48**: 499-504.

Keith I, Day R, Lemaire S, & Lemaire I (1987) Asbestos-induced fibrosis in rats: increase in lung mast cells and autocoid contents. Exp Lung Res, **13**: 311-327.

Kenny LC (1984) Asbestos fibre counting by image analysis - the performance of the Manchester programme on Magiscan. Ann Occup Hyg, **28**: 401-415.

Kimizuka G, Wang NS, & Hayashi Y (1987) Physical and microchemical alterations of chrysotile and amosite asbestos in the hamster lung. J Toxicol Environ Health, **21**: 251-264.

Kimizuka G, Azuma M, Ishibashi M, Shinozaki K, & Hayashi Y (1993) Co-carcinogenic effect of chrysotile and amosite asbestos with benzo(a)pyrene in the lung of hamsters. Acta Pathol Jpn, **43**: 149-153.

Kimura K (1987) [Asbestos and environment.] Dig Sci Lab, **42**: 4-13 (in Japanese).

Kjuus H, Skaerven R, Langard S, Lien J, & Aamodt T (1986) A case-reference study of lung cancer, occupational exposures and smoking. Scand J Work Environ Health, **12**: 203-209.

Kobayashi H, Ming ZW, Watanabe H, & Ohnishi Y (1987) A quantitative study of the distribution of asbestos bodies in extrapulmonary organs. Acta Pathol Jpn, **37**(3): 375-83.

Kodama Y, Boreiko CJ, Mannes SC, & Hesterberg TW (1993) Cytotoxic and cytogenetic effects of asbestos on human bronchial epithelial cells in culture. Carcinogenesis, **14**: 691-697.

Kogan FM (1982) Changes in occupational morbidity among workers in the asbestos mining industry in relation to the improvement of working conditions. Arch Immunol Ther Exp, **30**: 277-283.

Kogan FM (1989) Re: Chrysotile asbestos and mesothelioma of the pleura. Am J Ind Med, **15**: 123.

Kogevinas M, Boffetta P, & Pearce N (1994) Occupational exposure to carcinogens in developing countries. In: Pearce N, Matos E, Vainio H, Boffetta P, & Kogevinas M ed. Occupational cancer in developing countries. Lyon, International Agency for Research on Cancer, pp 63-95 (IARC Scientific Publications No. 129).

Kohyama N (1989) Airborne asbestos levels in non-occupational environments in Japan. In: Bignon J, Peto J, & Saracci J ed. Non-occupational exposure to mineral fibres. Lyon, International Agency for Research on Cancer, pp 262-276 (IARC Scientific Publications No. 90).

Kohyama N & Suzuki Y (1991) Analysis of asbestos fibres in lung parenchyma, pleural plaques and mesothelioma tissues of North American insulation workers. Ann NY Acad Sci, **643**: 27-52.

Korkina LG, Durnev AD, Suslova TB, Cheremisina ZP, Daugel-Dauge NO, & Afanas'ev IB (1992) Oxygen radical-mediated mutagenic effect of asbestos on human lymphocytes: suppression by oxygen radical scavengers. Mutat Res, **265**: 245-253.

Koshi K, Kohyama N, Myojo T, & Fukuda K (1991) Cell toxicity, hemolytic action and clastogenic activity of asbestos and its substitutes. Ind Health, **29**: 37-56.

Kouzan S, Brody AR, Nettesheim P, & Eling T (1985) Production of arachidonic acid metabolites by macrophages exposed in vitro to asbestos, carbonyl iron particles, or calcium ionophore. Am Rev Respir Dis, **131**: 624-632.

La Vecchia C, Lucchini F, Negri E, Boyle P, Maisonneuve P, & Levi F (1992) Trends of cancer mortality in Europe, 1955-1989: II. Respiratory tract, bone, connective and soft tissue sarcomas, and skin. Eur J Cancer, **28**: 514-599.

Landesman JM & Mossman BT (1982) Induction of ornithine decarboxylase in hamster tracheal epithelial cells exposed to asbestos and 12-o-tetradecanoylphorbol-13-acetate. Cancer Res, **42**: 3669-3675.

Langer AM & McCaughey WTM (1982) Mesothelioma in a brake repair worker. Lancet, **2**: 1101-1102.

Langer AM & Nolan RP (1986) The properties of chrysotile as determinants of biological activity. In: Wagner C ed. The biological effects of chrysotile. Accomplished Oncol, **1**: 30-51.

Langer AM & Nolan RP (1994) Chrysotile: its occurrence and properties as variables controlling biological effects. Ann Occup Hyg, **38**: 427-451.

Langer AM & Pooley FD (1973) Identification of single asbestos fibers in human tissue. In: Bogovski P, Gilson JC, Timbrell V, & Wagner JC ed. Biological effects of asbestos. Lyon, International Agency for Research on Cancer, pp 199-125 (IARC Scientific Publication No. 8).

References

Langer AM, Rubin I, & Selikoff IJ (1970) Electron microprobe analysis of asbestos bodies. In: Shapiro A ed. Proceedings of the International Conference on Pneumoconiosis, Johannesburg, 1969. Cape Town, Oxford University Press, pp 57-69.

Lauth J & Schurr K (1983) Some effects of chrysotile asbestos on a planktonic alga (*Cryptomonas erosa*). Micron Microsc Acta, **14**: 93-94.

Lauth J & Schurr K (1984) Entry of chrysotile asbestos fibres from water into the planktonic alga (*Cryptomonas erosa*). Micron Microsc Acta, **15**: 113-114.

Le Bouffant L, Daniel H, Henin JP, & Martin JC (1985) Carcinogenic potency of chrysotile fibres of the length < 5 um. Cah Notes Doc, **118**: 83-89.

Le Bouffant L, Daniel H, Henin JP, Martin JC, Normand C, Tichoux G, & Trolard F (1987) Experimental study on the long-term effects of inhaled MMMF on the lungs of rats. Ann Occup Hyg, **31**: 765-790.

Le Gven JMM, Ogden TL, Shenton-Taylor T, & Verrill JF (1984) The HSE/NPL phase contrast test slide. Ann Occup Hyg, **28**: 237-247.

Leanderson P, Soederkvist P, Tagesson C, & Axelson O (1988) Formation of 8-hydroxydeoxyguanosine by asbestos and man-made mineral fibres. Br J Ind Med, **45**: 309-311.

Lebel J (1995a) Static sampling in the asbestos mines and mills of the members companies of Q.A.M.A. Sherbrooke, Quebec Asbestos Mining Association.

Lebel J (1995b) Review of fibre concentrations in Quebec asbestos mining towns. Sherbrooke, Quebec Asbestos Mining Association.

Lechner JF, Tokiwa T, & La Vek M (1985) Asbestos-associated chromosomal changes in human mesothelial cells. Proc Natl Acad Sci (USA), **82**: 3884-3888.

Lee RJ, Van Orden DR, Com M, & Crump KS (1992) Exposure to airborne asbestos in buildings. Regul Toxicol Pharmacol, **16**: 93-98.

Lemaire I (1985) Characterization of the bronchoalveolar cellular response in experimental asbestosis: Different reactions depending on the fibrogenic potential. Am Rev Respir Dis, **131**: 144-149.

Lemaire I (1991) Selective differences in macrophage populations and monokine production in resolving pulmonary granuloma and fibrosis. Am J Pathol, **138**: 487-495.

Lemaire I, Nadeau D, Dunnigan J, & Masse S (1985) An assessment of the fibrogenic potential of very short 4T30 chrysotile by intratracheal instillation in rats. Environ Res, **36**: 314-326.

Lemaire I, Dubois C, Grondin C, & Gingras D (1986a) Immunoregulation of lung fibroblast growth: alteration in asbestos-induced pulmonary fibrosis. Clin Exp Immunol, **66**: 201-208.

Lemaire I, Gingras D, & Lemaire S (1986b) Effects of chrysotile asbestos on DNA synthesis and growth of human embryonic lung fibroblasts. J Environ Pathol Toxicol Oncol, **6**: 169-180.

Lemaire I, Beaudoin H, Masse S, & Girondin C (1986c) Alveolar macrophage stimulation of lung fibroblast growth in asbestos induced pulmonary fibrosis. Am J Pathol, **122**: 205-211.

Lemaire I, Beaudoin H, & Dubois C (1986d) Cytokine regulation of lung fibroblast proliferation: Pulmonary and systematic changes in asbestos induced pulmonary fibrosis. Am Rev Respir Dis, **134**: 653-658.

Lemaire I, Dionne PG, Nadeau D, & Dunnigan J (1989) Rat lung reactivity to natural and man-made fibrous silicates following short-term exposure. Environ Res, **48**: 193-210.

Li AP (1986) *In vitro* lung epithelial cell system for evaluating the potential toxicity of inhalable materials. Food Chem Toxicol, **24**: 527-534.

Liddell FDK (1994) Cancer mortality in chrysotile mining and milling: exposure-response. Ann Occup Hyg, **38**: 519-523.

Liddell FDK, Gibbs GW, & McDonald JC (1982) Radiological changes and fibre exposure in chrysotile workers aged 60-69 years at Thetford Mines. Ann Occup Hyg, **26**: 889-898.

Lippmann M, Yeates DB, & Albert RE (1980) Deposition, retention and clearance of inhaled particles. Br J Ind Med, **37**: 337-362.

Litistorf G, Guillemin M, Buffat P, & Iselin F (1985) Ambient air pollution by mineral fibers in Switzerland. Staub-Reinhalt Luft, **45**: 302-307.

Livingston GK, Rom WN, & Morris MV (1980) Asbestos-induced sister chromatid exchanges in cultured Chinese hamster ovarian fibroblast cells. J. Environ Pathol Toxicol, **4**: 373-82.

Lorimer WV, Rohl AN, & Miller A (1976) Asbestos exposure in brake repair workers in the United States. Mt Sinai J Med, **43**: 207-218.

Lu Y-P, Lasne C, Lowy R, & Chouroulinkov I (1988) Use of the orthogonal design method to study the synergistic effects of asbestos fibres and 12-*o*-tetradecanoylphorbol-13-acetate (TPA) in the BALB/3T3 cell transformation system. Mutagenesis, **3**: 355-362.

Lund LG & Aust AE (1991) Iron-catalyzed reactions may be responsible for the biochemical and biological effects of asbestos. BioFactors, **3**: 83-89.

Lynch J (1968) Brake lining decomposition products. J Am Pollut Control Assoc, **18**: 824-826.

Lynch JR & Ayer HE (1966) Measurement of dust exposures in the asbestos textile industry. Am Ind Hyg Assoc J, **27**: 431-437.

McClellan RO, Miller FJ, Hesterberg TW, Warheit DB, Bunn WB, Dement JM, Kane AB, Lippmann M, Mast RW, McConnell EE, & Reinhardt CF (1992) Approaches to evaluating the toxicity and carcinogenicity of man-made fibres. Regul Toxicol Pharmacol, **16(3)**: 321-364.

McConnell EE (1982) NIEHS carcinogenesis bioassays of chrysotile asbestos in Syrian golden hamsters: Workshop on Ingested Asbestos - Summary. Cincinnati, Ohio, US Environmental Protection Agency, Health Research Laboratory.

McConnell EE, Shefner AM, Rust JH, & Moore JA (1983) Chronic effects of dietary exposure to amosite and chrysotile asbestos in Syrian Golden hamsters. Environ Health Perspect, **53**: 11-25.

McCrone WC (1978) Identification of asbestos by polarized light microscopy. Gaithersburg, Maryland, US National Bureau of Standards, pp 235-248 (Special Publication 506).

References

McCrone (1991) Data provided to the literature review panel, HEI-AR. Norcross, Georgia, McCrone Environmental Services Inc.

McDermott M, Bevan MM, Elmes PC, Allardyce JT, & Bradley AC (1982) Lung function and radiographic change in chrysotile workers in Swaziland. Br J Ind Med, **39**: 338-343.

McDonald AD & McDonald JC (1980) Malignant mesothelioma in North America. Cancer, **46**: 1650-1656.

McDonald JC & McDonald AD (1993) Re: Work-related mesothelioma in Quebec. Am J Ind Med, **24**: 245-246.

McDonald JC, Becklake MR, Gibbs GW, McDonald AD, & Rossiter CE (1974) The health of chrysotile mine and mill workers of Quebec. Arch Environ Health, **28**: 61-68.

McDonald JC, Liddell FDK, Gibbs GW, Eyssen GE, & McDonald AD (1980) Dust exposure and mortality in chrysotile mining, 1910-75. Br J Ind Med, **37**: 11-24.

McDonald AD, Fry JS, Woolley AJ, & McDonald JC (1983a) Dust exposure and mortality in an American chrysotile textile plant. Br J Ind Med, **40**: 361-367.

McDonald AD, Fry JS, Woolley AJ, & McDonald JC (1983b) Dust exposure and mortality in an American factory using chrysotile, amosite, and crocidolite in mainly textile manufacture. Br J Ind Med, **40**: 368-374.

McDonald AD, Fry JS, Woolley AJ, & McDonald JC (1984) Dust exposure and mortality in an American chrysotile asbestos friction products plant. Br J Ind Med, **41**: 151-157.

McDonald AD, Liddell FDK, & McDonald JC (1992) Malignant mesothelioma in Quebec chrysotile miners and millers: a preliminary report. In: Proceedings of the Ninth International Symposium on Epidemiology in Occupational Health. Cincinnati, Ohio, National Institute of Occupational Safety and Health.

McDonald JC, Liddell FDK, Dufresne A, & McDonald AD (1993) The 1891-1920 birth cohort of Quebec chrysotile miners and millers: mortality 1976-88. Br J Ind Med, **50**: 1073-1081.

McDonald AD, Liddell FDK, & McDonald JC (1994) Malignant mesothelioma in Quebec chrysotile miners and millers: A preliminary report. In: Proceedings of the 9th International Symposium on Epidemiology in Occupational Health. Cincinnati, Ohio, National Institute of Occupational Safety and Health.

McGavran PD, Moore LB, & Brody AR (1990) Inhalation of chrysotile asbestos induced rapid cellular proliferation in small pulmonary vessels of mice and rats. Am J Pathol, **136**: 695-703.

Magnani C, Terracini G, Bertolone GP, Castaneto B, Cocito V, De Giovanni D, Paglieri P, & Botta M (1987) [Mortality from cancer and other diseases of respiratory tract among asbestos-cement workers in Casale Monferrato: historical cohort study.] Med Lav, **6**: 441-453 (in Italian).

Mancuso TF (1988) Relative risk of mesothelioma among railroad workers exposed to chrysotile. Am J Ind Med, **13**: 639-657.

Marsh JP & Mossman BT (1988) Mechanisms of induction of ornithine decarboxylase activity in tracheal epithelial cells by asbestiform minerals. Cancer Res, **48**: 709-714.

Marsh JP & Mossman BT (1991) Role of asbestos and active oxygen species in activation and expression of ornithine decarboxylase in hamster tracheal epithelial cells. Cancer Res, 51: 167-173.

Menichini E & Marconi A (1982) [Asbestos in brake and clutch factories: Results of an environmental survey.] G Ital Med Lav, 4: 197-202 (in Italian).

Middleton AP (1982) Analysis of airborne dust samples for chrysotile by x-ray diffraction. Ann Occup Hyg, 25: 443-447.

Middleton AP, Beckett ST, & Davis JMG (1979) Further observations on the short-term retention and clearance of asbestos in rats, using UICC reference samples. Ann Occup Hyg, 22: 141-152.

Mikalsen SO, Rivedal E, & Sanner T (1988) Morphological transformation of Syrian hamster embryo cells induced by mineral fibres and the alleged enhancement of benzo/a/pyrene. Carcinogenesis, 9: 891-899.

Millette JR ed. (1983) Summary Workshop on Ingested Asbestos. Environ Health Perspect, 53: 1-204.

Millette JR, Clark PJ, Pansing FM, & Twyman JD (1980) Concentration and size of asbestos in water supplies. Environ Health Perspect, 34: 13-25.

Minne E, Lenelle Y, Derouane A, & Verduyn G (1991) Survey of the environmental airborne fiber exposure by transmission electron microscopy. In: Proceedings of the AIA/NIOH International Colloquium on Dust Measurement Techniques and Strategy. Budapest, National Institute of Occupational Health, pp 152-163.

Monchaux G, Bignon J, Jaurand MC, Lafuma J, Sebastien P, Masse R, Hirsch A, & Goni J (1981) Mesotheliomas in rats following inoculation with acid-leached chrysotile asbestos and other mineral fibres. Carcinogenesis, 2: 229-236.

Moore LL (1988) Asbestos exposure associated with automotive brake repair in Pennsylvania. Am Ind Hyg Assoc J, 49: A12-A13.

Morgan A (1994) The removal of fibres of chrysotile asbestos from lung. Ann Occup Hyg, 38: 643-646.

Morgan A & Cralley LJ (1973) Chemical characteristics of asbestos and associated trace elements. In: Bogovski P, Gilson JC, Timbrell V, & Wagner JC ed. Biological effects of mineral fibres. Lyon, International Agency for Research on Cancer, pp 113-118 (IARC Scientific Publication No. 8).

Morgan A, Evans JC, & Holmes A (1977) Deposition and clearance of inhaled fibrous minerals in the rat: Studies using radioactive tracer technique. In: Walton HW ed. Inhaled particles IV - Part I. Proceedings of an International Symposium, Edinburgh, 1975. Oxford, Pergamon Press, pp 259-272.

Mossman BT & Begin RO ed.(1989) Effects of mineral dusts on cells. Berlin, Heidelberg, New York, Springer-Verlag, 470 pp (NATO ASI Series H. Cell Biology, Volume 30)..

Mossman BT & Sesko AM (1990) In vitro assays to predict the pathogenicity of mineral fibers. Toxicology, 60: 53-61.

References

Mossman BT, Bignon J, Corn M, Seaton A, & Gee JBL (1990) Asbestos: Scientific developments and implications for public policy. Science, **247**: 294-301.

Muhle H, Spurny K, & Pott F (1983) [Inhalation experiments on retention, lung clearance, and migration of asbestos and glass fibres in dependence of cigarette smoking.] VDR-Bericht, **475**: 247-251 (in German).

Muhle E, Pott F, Bellmann B, Takenada S, & Ziem V (1987) Inhalation and injection experiments in rats to test the carcinogenicity of MMF. Ann Occup Hyg, **31**: 755-764.

Mukherjee AK, Rajmohan HR, Dave SK, Rajan BK, Kakde Y, & Raghavedra Rao S (1992) An environmental survey in chrysotile asbestos milling processes in India. Am J Ind Med, **22**: 543-551.

Nagy B & Bates TF (1952) Stability of chrysotile asbestos. Am Mineral Rev Mineralogy, **37**: 1055-1058.

Neuberger M & Kundi M (1990) Individual asbestos exposure: smoking and mortality - a cohort study in the asbestos cement industry. Br J Ind Med, **47**: 615-620.

Neuberger M & Kundi M (1993) Cancer in asbestos cement production and implication for risk management. In: Proceedings of the 24th Congress of the International Commission on Occupational Health, Nice, 26 September-1 October 1993. International Commission on Occupational Health and French Ministry of Labour, Employment and Professional Training.

Neuberger M, Frank W, Golob P, & Warbichler P (1996) [Asbestos concentrations in drinking water.] Zbl Hyg, **198**(4): 293-306 (in German).

Newhouse ML & Sullivan KR (1989) A mortality study of workers manufacturing friction materials: 1941-86. Br J Ind Med, **46**: 176- 179.

Nicholson WJ (1978) Chrysotile asbestos in air samples collected in Puerto Rico. Final Report to US Consumer Products Safety Commission on Contract (CPSC 77128000). New York, Mount Sinai School of Medicine, Environmental Sciences Laboratory.

Nicholson WJ (1988) Airborne levels of mineral fibers in the non-occupational environment. New York, Mount Sinai School of Medicine.

Nicholson WJ & Landrigan PJ (1994) The carcinogenicity of chrysotile asbestos. In: Mehlman MA ed. Advances in modern environmental toxicology, Volume XXII. Princeton, New Jersey, Princeton Scientific Publishing Company Inc, pp 407-423.

Nicholson WJ & Pundsack FL (1973) Asbestos in the environment. In: Biological effects of asbestos. Lyon, International Agency for Research on Cancer, pp 126-130.

Nicholson WJ, Selikoff IJ, Seidman H, Lilis R, & Formby P (1979) Long-term mortality experience of chrysotile miners and millers in Thetford Mines, Quebec. Ann NY Acad Sci, **330**: 11-21

NIOSH (1989a) Asbestos fibers - NIOSH method 7402. In: NIOSH manual of analytical methods, revision 1. Cincinnati, Ohio, National Institute of Occupational Safety and Health.

NIOSH (1989b) Asbestos bulk - NIOSH method 9002. In: NIOSH manual of analytical methods, revision 1. Cincinnati, Ohio, National Institute of Occupational Safety and Health.

NTP (1985) Toxicology and carcinogenesis studies of chrysotile asbestos in F344/N rats (feed study). Research Triangle Park, US Department of Health and Human Services, National Toxicology Program, 390 pp (Technical Report Series No. 295; NIH Publication No. 86-2551).

Oberdörster G (1994) Macrophage-associated responses to chrysotile. Ann Occup Hyg, **38**: 601-615.

Oberdörster G & Lehnert BA (1991) Toxicological aspects of the pathogenesis of fiber-induced pulmonary effects. In: Brown RC ed. Mechanisms in fibre carcinogenesis. New York, Plenum Press, pp 157-179.

Oberdörster G, Boose C, Pott F, & Pfeiffer U (1980) In vitro dissolution rates of trace elements from mineral fibres. In: Brown RC, Chamberlain M, Davies R, & Gormley P ed. New York, London, Academic Press, pp 183-189.

Oghiso Y, Kagan E, & Brody AR (1984) In pulmonary distribution of inhaled chrysotile and crocidolite asbestos: ultrastructural features. Br J Exp Pathol, **65**: 467-484.

Ohlson CG & Hogstedt C (1985) Lung cancer among asbestos cement workers. A Swedish cohort study and a review. Br J Ind Med, **42**: 397-402.

Olofsson K & Mark J (1989) Specificity of asbestos-induced chromosomal aberrations in short-term cultures of human mesothelial cells. Cancer Genet Cytogenet, **41**: 33-39.

OPCS/HSE (1995) In: Drever F ed. Occupational health decenial supplement No 10. London, Office of Population Censuses and Surveys, Health and Safety Executive, pp 136-152.

Osgood C & Sterling D (1991) Chrysotile and amosite asbestos induce germ-line aneuploidy in Drosophila. Mutat Res, **261**: 9-13.

Palekar LD, Eyre JF, Most BM, & Coffin DL (1987) Metaphase and anaphase analysis of V79 cells exposed to erionite, UICC chrysotile and UICC crocidolite. Carcinogenesis, **8**: 553-560.

Parnes S (1990) Asbestos and cancer of the larynx: is there a relationship? Laryngoscope, **100**: 254-261.

Parsons RC, Bryant DG, & Edstrom HW (1986) Variation in fibre and dust counts in an asbestos mine and mill. Ann Occup Hyg, **30**: 63-75.

Paterour MJ, Bignon J, & Jaurand MC (1985) In vitro transformation of rat pleural mesothelial cells by chrysotile fibres and/or benzo/a/pyrene. Carcinogenesis, **6**: 523-529.

Pelin K, Husgafvel-Pursiainen K, Vallas M, Vanhala E, & Linnainmaa K (1992) Cytotoxicity and anaphase aberrations induced by mineral fibres in cultured human mesothelial cells. Toxic in Vitro, **6**: 445-450.

Perkins RC, Scheule RK, Hamilton R, Gomez G, Freidman G, & Holian A (1993) Human alveolar macrophage cytokine release in response to in vitro and in vivo asbestos exposure. Exp Lung Res, **19**: 55-65.

Peto J (1980) Lung cancer mortality in relation to measured dust levels in an asbestos textile factory. In: Wagner JC ed. Biological effects of mineral fibres. Lyon, International Agency for Research on Cancer, pp 829-836 (IARC Scientific Publications No. 30).

References

Peto J (1989) Fibre carcinogenesis and environmental hazards. In: Bignon J, Peto J, & Saracci R ed. Non-occupational exposure to mineral fibres. Lyon, International Agency on Research for Cancer, pp 457-470 (IARC Scientific Publications No. 90).

Peto J, Doll R, Hermon C, Binns W, Clayton R, & Goffe T (1985) Relationship of mortality to measures of environmental asbestos pollution in an asbestos textile factory. Ann Occup Hyg, 29: 305-355.

Peto J, Hodgson JT, Matthews FE, & Jones JR (1995) Continuing increase in mesothelioma mortality in Britain. Lancet, 345: 535-539.

Petruska JM, Marsh J, Bergeron M, & Mossman BT (1990) Brief inhalation of asbestos compromises superoxide production in cells from bronchoalveolar lavage. Am J Respir Cell Mol Biol, 2: 129-136.

Pigg BJ (1994) The uses of chrysotile. Ann Occup Hyg, 38: 453-458.

Pinkerton KE & Yu CP (1988) Intrapulmonary airway branching and parenchymal deposition of chrysotile asbestos fibres. In: Wehner AP & Felton DL ed. Proceeding of an International Symposium on Interaction of Inhaled Mineral Fibres and Cigarette Smoke. Seattle, Washington, Battell Press, pp 211-222.

Pinkerton KE, Plopper CG, Mercer RR, Roggli VL, Patra AL, Brody AR, & Crapo JD (1986) Airway branching patterns influence asbestos fiber location and the extent of tissue injury in the pulmonary parenchyma. Lab Invest, 55: 688-695.

Pinkerton KE, Young SL, Fram EK, & Crapo JD (1990) Alveolar type II cell responses to chronic inhalation of chrysotile asbestos in rats. Am J Respir Cell Mol Biol, 3: 543-552.

Piolatto G, Negri E, La Veccia C, Pira E, Decarli A, & Peto J (1990) An update of cancer mortality among chrysotile asbestos miners in Balangero, Northern Italy. Br J Ind Med, 47: 810-814.

Platek SF, Groth DH, Ulrich CE, Stettler LF, Finnell MS, & Stoll M (1985) Chronic inhalation of short asbestos fibres. Fundam Appl Toxicol, 5: 327-340.

Polissar NL (1993) Asbestos in drinking water: health issues. In: Gibbs GW, Dunnigan J, Kido K, & Higashi T ed. Health risks from exposure to mineral fibres - An international perspective. North York, Captus University Publications, pp 164-182.

Pooley FD (1987) In: Antman K & Aisner J ed. Asbestos mineralogy. Orlando, Florida, Grune and Stratton Inc, pp 3-27.

Pott F (1978) Some aspects on the dosimetry of the carcinogenic potency of asbestos and other fibrous dusts. Staub-Reinhalt Luft, 38: 486-490.

Pott F (1994) Asbestos use and carcinogenicity in Germany and a comparison with animal studies. Ann Occup Hyg, 38: 589-600.

Pott F & Friedrichs KH (1972) Tumours in rats after intraperitoneal injection of asbestos dusts. Naturwissenschaften, 59: 318- 332.

Pott F, Huth F, & Friederichs KH (1972) [Tumors of rats after i.p. injection of powdered chrysotile and benzo(a)pyrene.] Zentralbl Bakteriolt Orig B, 155(5): 463-469 (in German).

Pott F, Friedrichs KH, & Huth F (1976) [Results of animals experiments concerning the carcinogenic effect of fibrous dusts and their interpretation in regard to the carcinogenesis in humans.] Zentbl Bakteriol Hyg I. Abt Orig B, **162**: 467-505 (in German).

Pott F, Ziem V, Reiffer KJ, Huth F, Ernst H, & Mohr V (1987) Carcinogenicity studies on fibres, metal compounds and some other dusts in rats. Exp Pathol, **32**: 129-152.

Pott F, Roller M, Ziem U, Reiffer FJ, Bellmann B, Rosenbruch M, & Huth F (1989) Carcinogenicity studies on natural and man-made fibres with the intraperitoneal test in rats. In: Bignon J, Peto J, & Saracci R ed. Non-occupational exposure to mineral fibres. Lyon, International Agency for Research on Cancer, pp 173-179 (IARC Scientific Publication No. 90).

Price B, Crump KS, & Baird EC (1992) Airborne asbestos levels in buildings: maintenance workers and occupant exposures. J Exp Anal Environ Epidemiol, **2**: 357-373.

Proctor J & Woodall SRJ (1975) The ecology of serpentine soils. Adv Ecol Res, **9**: 255-366.

Raffn E, Lynge E, Juel K, & Korsgaard B (1989) Incidence of cancer and mortality among employees in the asbestos cement industry in Denmark. Br J Ind Med, **46**: 90-96.

Rendall REG (1970) The data sheets on the chemical and physical properties of the UICC standard reference samples. In: Shapiro H ed. Proceedings of the International Pneumoconiosis Conference. New York, Pergamon Press, pp 23-77.

Rickards AL (1973) Estimation of submicrogram quantities of chrysotile asbestos by electron microscopy. Anal Chem, **45**: 809-811.

Rickards AL (1991) AIA activities and the future use of fibres. Proceedings of the AIA/NIOH International Colloquium on Dust Measurement Techniques and Strategy. Budapest, National Institute of Occupational Health, pp 62-73.

Rickards AL (1994) Levels of workplace exposure. Ann Occup Hyg, **38**: 469-475.

Rita P & Reddi PP (1986) Effect of chrysotile asbestos fibres on germ cells of mice. Environ Res, **41**: 139-143.

Ritter-Studnicka H (1970) [The flora of serpentines in Bosnia.] Bibl Bot, **130**: 1-100 (in German).

Roberts BA & Proctor J ed. (1993) The ecology of areas with serpentinized rocks: A world view. Amsterdam, Kluver Academic Publishers, 420 pp.

Rodelsperger K, Jahn H, Bruckel B, Manke J, Paur R, & Woitowitz HJ (1986) Asbestos dust exposure during brake repair. Am J Ind Med, **10**: 63-72.

Roesler JA, Woitowitz HJ, Lange HJ, Ulm K, Woitowitz RH, & Roedelsperger K (1993) [Effects of occupational asbestos exposure and malignant tumor mortality in Germany: Standardized proportional mortality in high risk groups - Research Report Asbestos IV.] St Augustin, General Federation of Commercial Employment Accident Funds (in German).

Rogers AJ, Leigh J, Berry G, Ferguson DA, Mulder HB, & Ackad M (1991a) Relationship between lung asbestos fibre type and concentration and relative risk of mesothelioma - a case-control study. Cancer, **67**: 1912-1920.

Rogers AJ, Leigh J, Berry G, Ferguson DA, Mulder HB, Ackad M, & Morgan GG (1991b) Dose-response relationship between airborne and lung asbestos fibre type, length and concentration of the relative risk of mesothelioma. In: McCallum I ed. Proceedings of the 7th BOHS Inhaled Particles Symposium, Edinburgh, 1991.

Roggli VL & Brody AR (1984) Changes in numbers and dimension of chrysotile asbestos fibres in lungs of rats following short-term exposure. Exp Lung Res, 7: 133-147.

Rohl AN, Langer AM, Wolff MS, & Weisman I (1976) Asbestos exposure during brake lining maintenance and repair. Environ Res, 12: 110-128.

Rohl AN, Langer AM, Klimentidis R, Wolff A, & Selikoff IJ (1977) Asbestos content of dust encountered in brake maintenance and repair. Proc R Soc Med, 70: 32-37.

Rom WN & Paakko P (1991) Activated alveolar macrophages express the insulin-like growth factor-I receptor. Am J Respir Cell Mol Biol, 4: 432-439.

Rood AP (1991) Fibres in the general environment. In: Liddell D & Miller K ed. Mineral fibres and health. Boca Raton, Florida, CRC Press, pp 93-102.

Rooker SJ, Vaughan NP, & Le Guen JM (1982) On the visibility of fibers by phase contrast microscopy. Am Ind Hyg Assoc J, 43: 505-515.

Rowlands N, Gibbs GW, & McDonald AD (1982) Asbestos fibres in the lungs of chrysotile miners and millers - A preliminary report. Ann Occup Hyg, 26(1-4): 411-415.

Rowson DM (1978) The chrysotile content of the wear debris of brake lining. Wear, 47: 315-321.

Rubino GF, Newhouse ML, Murray R, Scansetti G, Piolatto G, & Aresini GA (1979a) Radiologic changes after cessation of exposure among chrysotile asbestos miners in Italy. Ann NY Acad Sci, 330: 157-161.

Rubino GF, Piolatto G, Newhouse ML, Scansetti G, Aresini GA, & Murray R (1979b) Mortality of chrysotile asbestos workers at the Balangero Mine, Northern Italy. Br J Ind Med, 36: 187-194.

Ruhe RL & Lipscomb J (1985) Health hazard evaluation report 84-151-1544. Cincinnati, Ohio, National Institute of Occupational Safety and Health.

Sawyer RN (1977) Asbestos exposure in a Yale building. Environ Res, 13: 146-169.

Schapira RM, Osornio-Vargas AR, & Brody AR (1991) Inorganic particles induce secretion of a macrophage homologue of platelet-derived growth factor in a density-and time-dependent manner in vitro. Exp Lung Res, 17: 1011-1024.

Schreier H (1987) Asbestos fibers introduce trace metals into streamwater and sediments. Environ Pollut, 43: 229-242.

Schreier H (1989) Asbestos in the natural environment. Amsterdam, Oxford, New York, Elsevier Science Publishers, 159 pp (Studies in Environmental Sciences, Volume 37).

Schreier H & Timmenga H (1986) Earthwork response to asbestos-rich serpentinitic sediments. Soil Biol Biochem, 1: 85-89.

Schreier H, Shelford JA, & Nguhyen TD (1986) Asbestos fibers and trace metals in the blood of cattle grazing in fields inundated by asbestos-rich sediments. Environ Res, 41: 95-109.

Schreier H, Omueti JA, & Lavkulich LM (1987a) Weathering processes of asbestos-rich serpentinitic sediments. Soil Sci Soc Am J, 51: 993-999.

Schreier H, Northcote T, & Hall K (1987b) Trace metals in fish exposed to asbestos-rich sediments. Water Air Soil Pollut, 35: 279-291.

Sebastien P, Janson X, Gaudichet A, Hirsch A, & Bignon J (1980) Asbestos retention in human respiratory tissues: comparative measurements in lung parenchyma and in parietal pleura. In: Wagner J ed. Biological effects of mineral fibres. Lyon, International Agency for Research on Cancer, pp 237-246 (IARC Scientific Publications No. 30).

Sebastien P, Plourde M, & Robb R (1986a) Ambient air asbestos survey in Quebec mining towns. Part 2 - Main study. Ottawa, Environment Canada (Report 5/AP/RQ-2E).

Sebastien P, Begin R, Case BW, & McDonald JC (1986b) Inhalation of chrysotile dust. In: Wagner JC ed. The biological effects of chrysotile. Philadelphia, Pennsylvania, JB Lippincott, pp 19-29.

Sebastien P, McDonald JC, McDonald AD, Case B, & Harley R (1989) Respiratory cancer in chrysotile textile and mining industries: exposure inferences from lung analysis. Br J Ind Med, 46: 180-187.

Sebastien P, Begin R, & Masse S (1990) Mass, number and size of lung fibres in the pathogenesis of asbestosis in sheep. Int J Exp Pathol, 71: 1-10.

Seshan K (1983) How are the physical and chemical properties of chrysotile asbestos altered by a 10-year residence in water and up to 5 days in simulated stomach acid? Environ Health Perspect, 53: 143-148.

Sheehy JW, Godbey FW, Cooper TC, Lenichan KN, & Van Wagenen HD (1987) In-depth survey report: control technology for brake drum service operations at Ohio Department of Transportations Maintenance Facility. Washington, DC, Government Reports Announcements & Index (Issue 16).

Shride AF (1973) Asbestos. In: Probst D & Pratt W ed. US mineral resources. Washington, DC, US Department of the Interior, pp 63-72.

Siemiatycki J (1991) Risk factors for cancer in the workplace. Boca Raton, Florida, CRC Press.

Sincock AM, Delhanty JD, & Casey GA (1982) A comparison of the cytogenetic response to asbestos and glass fibres in CHO cell lines. Mutat Res, 101, 257-268.

Skidmore JW & Dufficy BL (1983) Environmental history of a factory producing friction material. Br J Ind Med, 40: 8-12.

Skikne MI, Talbot JH, & Rendall RW (1971) Electron diffraction patterns of UICC asbestos samples. Environ Res, 4: 141-145.

Skinner HCW, Ross M, & Frondel C (1988) Asbestos and other fibrous materials. New York, Oxford University Press, pp 29-33.

References

Smith WE, Hubert DD, Miller L, Badollet MS, & Churg J (1968) Tests for levels of carcinogenicity of asbestos. In: Proceedings of the International Conference on Biological Effects of Asbestos. Berlin, German Central Institute for Occupational Health, pp 240-242.

Speil S & Leineweber JP (1969) Asbestos minerals in modern technology. Environ Res, 2: 166-208.

Spurny KR (1982) On the problem of measuring and analysis of chemically changed mineral fibres in the environment and in biological materials. Sci Total Environ, 23: 239-249.

Stanton MF & Wrench C (1972) Mechanisms of mesothelioma induction with asbestos and fibrous glass. J Natl Cancer Inst, 48: 797-821.

Stanton MF, Layard M, Tegeris A, Miller M, & Kent E (1977) Carcinogenicity of fibrous glass: pleural response in the rat in relation to fibre dimension. J Natl Cancer Inst, 58: 587-603.

Sturm W, Menze B, Krause J, & Thriene B (1994) Use of asbestos, health risks and induced occupational diseases in the former East Germany. Toxicol Lett, 72: 317-324.

Szeszenia-Dabrowska N, Wilczynska U, & Szumczak W (1988) A mortality study among male workers occupationally exposed to asbestos dust in Poland. Pol J Occup Med, 1: 77-87.

Teta MJ, Lewinsohn HC, Meigs JW, Vidone RA, Mowad LZ, & Flannery JT (1983) Mesothelioma in Connecticut, 1955-1979. Occupational and Geographic Association. J Occup Med, 25(10): 749-755.

Thomas HF, Benjamin IT, Elwood PC, & Sweetnam PM (1982) Further follow-up study of workers from an asbestos cement factory. Br J Ind Med, 39: 273-276.

Thornton I (1981) Geochemical aspects of the distribution and forms of heavy metals in soils. In: Lepp NW ed. Effect of heavy metal pollution on plants. London, New Jersey, Applied Science Publishers, vol 2, pp 1-33.

Tilkes F & Beck EG (1989) Cytotoxicity and carcinogenicity of chrysotile fibres from asbestos-cement production. In: Bignon J, Peto J, & Sarracci R ed. Non-occupational exposure to mineral fibres. Lyon, International Agency for Research on Cancer, pp 190-196 (IARC Scientific Publications No. 90).

Timbrell V (1965) The inhalation of fibrous dusts. Ann NY Acad Sci, 132: 255-273.

Timbrell V (1970) The inhalation of fibres. In: Shapiro HA ed. Proceedings of the International Pneumoconiosis Conference. New York, Pergamon Press, pp 3-9.

Timbrell V (1973) Physical factors as etiological mechanisms. In: Bogovski P, Gilson JC, Timbrell V, & Wagner JC ed. Biological effects of asbestos. Lyon, International Agency for Research on Cancer, pp 295-303 (IARC Scientific Publications No. 30).

Timbrell V (1975) Alignment of respirable asbestos fibres by magnetic fields. Ann Occup Hyg, 18: 299-311.

Timbrell V, Gilson JC, & Webster I (1968) UICC Standard reference samples of asbestos. Int J Cancer, 3: 406-408.

Toft P, Meek ME, Wigle DT, & Meranger JD (1984) Asbestos in drinking water. In: CRC critical reviews in environmental control. Ottawa, Department of National Health and Welfare, Health Protection Branch.

Tolbert PE, Eisen EA, Pothier LJ, Monson RR, Hallock MF, & Smith TJ (1992) Mortality studies of machining-fluid exposure in the automobile industry. Scand J Work Environ Health, **18**: 351-360.

Toyokuni S & Sagripanti JL (1993) Induction of oxidative single- and double-strand breaks in DNA by ferric citrate. Free Radiat Biol Med, **15**: 117-123.

Truhaut R & Chouroulinkov I (1989) Effect of long term ingestion of asbestos fibres in rats. In: Bignon J, Peto J, & Sarracci R ed. Non-occupational exposure to mineral fibres. Lyon, International Agency for Research on Cancer, pp 127-134 (IARC Scientific Publications No 90).

Tuckfield RC, Tsay Y, Margeson DP, Ogden J, Chesson J, Buer K, Constant PC, Bergman FJ, & Rose DP (1988) Final report for tasks 1-6: Evaluation of asbestos abatement techniques - Phase 3: Removals. Washington, DC, US Environmental Protection Agency (EPA-68-02-4294).

US Department of Interior (1986) Industrial minerals supply/demand data, 1974/1984 - Mineral industry surveys, April 18, 1986. Washington, DC, US Department of Interior.

US Department of Interior (1991) Asbestos: annual report. Washington, DC, US Department of Interior.

US Department of Interior (1993) Asbestos in 1992. Mineral Industry Surveys, April 23, 1993. Washington, DC, US Department of Interior.

US EPA (1980) Air quality criteria for sulfur oxides and particulates. Washington, DC, US Environmental Protection Agency, pp 11/28-11/32 (EPA-600/8-82-029c).

US EPA (1986) Airborne asbestos health assessment update, Washington, DC, US Environmental Protection Agency, 198 pp (EPA-600/8-84-003F).

US Occupational Safety and Health Administration (1986) Occupational exposure to asbestos, tremolite, anthophyllite, and actinolite: Final rules. Fed Ref, **29 CFR**: 22612-22790 (Parts 1910 and 1926).

US Occupational Safety and Health Administration (1994) Occupational exposure to asbestos. Fed Reg, **59**: 40964-41158.

Valić F (1993) Influence of exposure conversions and activity-specific exposure-response relationships on the chrysotile asbestos risk assessment. In: Gibbs GW, Dunnigan J, Kido M, & Higashi T ed. Health risks from exposure to mineral fibres. North York, Captus Press Inc, pp 129-135.

Valić F & Beritić-Stahuljak D (1993) Is chrysotile asbestos exposure a significant health risk to the general population? Cent Eur J Public Health, **1**: 26-30.

Valić F & Cigula M (1992) Interconvertibility of asbestos fibre count concentrations recorded by three most frequent methods. Arh hig rada toksikol, **43**: 359-364.

References

Van de Meeren A, Fleury J, Nebut M, Monchaux G, Janson X, & Jaurand M-C (1992) Mesothelioma in rats following intrapleural injection of chrysotile and phosphorylated chrysotile (chrysophosphate). Int J Cancer, **50**: 937-942.

Van Wagenen HD (1987) Preliminary survey report: Evaluation of brake drum service controls at Pennsylvania Bureau of Vehicle Management Harrisburg. Cincinnati, Ohio, National Institute of Occupational Safety and Health (Report CT-152-19a).

Verschaeve L, Palmer P, & In't Veld P (1985) On the uptake and genotoxicity of UICC Rhodesian chrysotile A in human primary lung fibroblasts. Naturwissenschaften, **72**: 326-327.

Viallat JR, Boutin C, Pietri JF, & Fondarai J (1983) Late progression of radiographic changes in Canari chrysotile mine and mill ex-workers. Arch Environ Health, **38**: 54-58.

Vincent JH, Johnston WB, Jones AD, & Johnston AM (1981) Static electrification of airborne asbestos: a study of its causes, assessment and effects on deposition in the lungs of rats. Am Ind Hyg Assoc J, **42**: 711-721.

Wagner JC (1962) Experimental production of mesothelial tumours of the pleura by implantation of dusts in laboratory animals. Nature (Lond), **196**: 180-181.

Wagner JC & Skidmore JW (1965) Asbestos dust deposition and retention in rats. Ann NY Acad Sci, **132**: 77-86.

Wagner JC, Berry G, & Timbrell V (1973) Mesotheliomata in rats after inoculation with asbestos and other minerals. Br J Cancer, **28**: 173-185.

Wagner JC, Berry G, Skidmore JW, & Timbrell V (1974) The effects of the inhalation of asbestos in rats. Br J Cancer, **29**: 252-269.

Wagner JC, Berry G, Skidmore JW, & Pooley FD (1980) The comparative effects of three chrysotiles by injection and inhalation in rats. In: Wagner JC ed. Biological effects of mineral fibres. Lyon, International Agency for Research on Cancer, pp 363-373 (IARC Scientific Publications No. 30).

Wagner JC, Berry G, & Pooley FD (1982) Mesotheliomas and asbestos type in asbestos textile workers. Br Med J, **285**: 606-606.

Wagner JC, Berry GB, Hill RJ, Munday DE, & Skidmore JW (1984) Animals experiments with MMM(V)F. Effects of inhalation and intraperitoneal inoculation in rats. In: Proceedings of a WHO/IARC Conference: Biological Effects of Man-Made Mineral Fibres. Copenhagen, World Health Organization, Regional Office for Europe, 209-233.

Walton NH (1982) The nature, hazards and assessment of occupational exposure to airborne asbestos dust: a review. Ann Occup Hyg, **25**(special issue): 117-247.

Wehner AP, Stuart BO, & Sanders CL (1979) Inhalation studies with Syrian golden hamsters. Proc Exp Tumor Res, **24**: 177.

Weill H, Rossiter CE, Waggenspack C, Jones RN, & Ziskind MM (1979) Differences in lung effects resulting from chrysotile and crocidolite exposure. In: Walton WH ed. Inhaled particles IV. Oxford, Pergamon Press, vol 2, pp 789-796.

Weiner R, Rees D, Lunga FJP, & Felix MA (1994) Third wave of asbestos-related disease from secondary use of asbestos. S Afr Med J, **84**: 158-160.

Weitzman SA & Graceffa P (1984) Asbestos catalyzes hydroxyl and superoxide radical generation from hydrogen peroxide. Arch Biochem, **228**: 373-376.

Weitzman SA & Weitberg AB (1985) Asbestos-catalysed lipid peroxidation and its inhibition by desferroxamine. Biochem J, **225**: 259-262.

White CD (1967) Absence of nodule formation on *Ceanothus cruneatu* in serpentine soils. Nature (Lond), **215**: 875.

WHO (1985) Reference methods for measuring airborne man-made mineral fibres (MMMF). Copenhagen, World Health Organization, Regional Office for Europe, pp 36-54.

WHO (1989) Occupational exposure limit for asbestos. Geneva, World Health Organization, Occupational Health (WHO/OCH 89.1).

WHO (1997) Determination of airborne fibre number concentrations: A recommended method by phase contrast optical microscopy. Geneva, World Health Organization. Occupational Health.

Wicks FJ (1979) Mineralogy, chemistry and crystallography of chrysotile asbestos. In: Ledoux RL ed. Short course in mineralogical techniques of asbestos determination. Ottawa, Mineralogical Association of Canada, pp 35-78.

Wild H (1975) Termites and serpentines of the Great Dyke of Rhodesia. Trans Rhod Sci Assoc, **57**: 1-11.

Wilkinson P, Hansell DM, Janssens J, Rubens M, Rudd RM, Newman Taylor A, & McDonald C (1995) Is lung cancer associated with asbestos exposure when there are no small opacities on the chest radiograph? Lancet, **345**: 1074-1078.

Williams RL & Muhlbaier JL (1982) Asbestos brake emissions. Environ Res, **29**: 70-82.

Wither ED & Brooks RR (1977) Hyperaccumulation of nickel by some plants of Southeast Asia. J Geochem Explor, **8**: 579-583.

Woitowitz HJ & Rodelsperger K (1991) Chrysotile asbestos and mesothelioma. Am J Ind Med, **19**: 551-553.

Woitowitz HJ & Rodelsperger K (1992) Chrysotile asbestos, mesothelioma and garage mechanics. Am J Ind Med, **21**: 453-455.

Woitowitz HJ & Rodelsperger K (1994) Mesothelioma among car mechanics? Ann Occup Hyg, **38**(4): 635-638.

Woodroofe HM (1956) Pyrolysis of chrysotile asbestos fibre. Trans Can Inst Min & Met, **59**: 363-368.

Wright A, Cowie H, Gormley IP, & Davis JMG (1986) The *in vitro* cytotoxicity of asbestos fibres: I.p388D1 cells. Am J Ind Med, **9**: 371-384.

References

Yada K (1967) Study of chrysotile asbestos by a high resolution electron microscope. Acta Cryst, **23**: 704-707.

Yang MY, Zhang JF, Fu B, Xu GH, Xu SL, Zhao XQ, Zhan QJ, & Zhao JD (1990) [Experimental study on incidence of pleural mesothelioma of rats caused by asbestos fibres of various length.] Chin J Ind Hyg Occup Dis, **8**: 292-294 (in Chinese).

Yegles M, Saint-Etienne L, Renier A, Janson X, & Jaurand MC (1993) Induction of metaphase and anaphase/telophase abnormalities by asbestos fibers in rat pleural mesothelial cells *in vitro*. Am J Respir Cell Mol Biol, **9**: 186-191.

Yoshimura H & Takemoto K (1991) [Effect of cigarette smoking and/or N-bis(2-hydrosypropyl)nitrosamine (PHPN) on the development of lung and pleural tumors in rats induced by administration of asbestos.] Jpn J Ind Health, **33**: 81-93 (in Japanese).

Zhu H & Wang Z (1993) Study of occupational lung cancer in asbestos factories in China. Br J Ind Med, **50**: 1039-1042.

Zou S, Wu Y, Ma F, Ma H, Sueng W, & Jiang Z (1990) Retrospective mortality study of asbestos workers in Laiyuan. In: Proceedings of the VIIth International Pneumoconiosis Conference. Pittsburgh, Ohio, Public Health Service, part II, pp 1242-1244 (Publication (NIOSH) No. 90-108).

1. RÉSUMÉ

1.1 Identité, propriétés physiques et chimiques, échantillonnage et analyse

Le chrysotile est un silicate de magnésium hydraté de structure fibreuse utilisé dans un grand nombre de produits du commerce. Il est très répandu aujourd'hui dans le commerce mondial. Les propriétés physiques et chimiques de ce minéral varient selon les différents gisements en exploitation. De nombreux minéraux accompagnent la fibre dans le minerai et parmi ceux-ci figurent sans doute certaines variétés d'amphibole fibreuse. On pense que la trémolite est particulièrement importante à cet égard; sa forme et sa concentration varient dans d'importantes proportions.

Du point de vue analytique, la recherche du chrysotile sur les lieux de travail oblige à recourir à la microscopie optique ou électronique. On a utilisé jusqu'ici divers instruments et dispositifs pour surveiller l'environnement en procédant à la recherche et au dosage des poussières et des fibres totales. Aujourd'hui, on utilise couramment la filtration sur membrane et le microscope à contraste de phase pour les mesures sur les lieux de travail (exprimées en nombre de fibres par ml d'air); on utilise aussi la microscopie électronique par transmission. Cette dernière technique est également employée pour l'analyse des prélèvements environnementaux. On a cherché à déterminer la charge tissulaire afin d'obtenir davantage de données sur l'exposition. En fonction du degré de détail que ces études on permis d'appréhender, on a pu en tirer des conclusions sur les mécanismes et les étiologies en cause.

On utilisait auparavant des techniques gravimétriques, la précipitation thermique ou la collecte sur mini-impacteur pour les contrôles sur les lieux de travail et ces mesures de poussières (et non pas de fibres) sont les seuls indices dont on dispose pour apprécier les relations exposition–réponse. Il y a eu de nombreuses tentatives en vue de convertir ces valeurs en nombres de fibre par volume d'air, mais elles n'ont rencontré qu'un succès très limité. On s'est rendu compte que les facteurs de conversion dépendaient du type d'industrie et

Résumé

même du type d'opération industrielle; les facteurs de conversion universels sont d'une grande variabilité.

1.2 Sources d'exposition professionnelle et environnementale

On trouve de faibles concentrations de chrysotile dans tout l'environnement de l'écorce terrestre (air, calottes glaciaires et sol). Les phénomènes naturels et les activités humaines contribuent à la production d'aérosols de fibres et à leur dissémination dans l'environnement. Parmi les sources d'origine humaine, on peut citer diverses activités professionnelles génératrices de poussières qui vont de l'extraction et du traitement du minerai jusqu'à la fabrication, aux applications, à l'utilisation et finalement, au rejet sous forme de déchets.

Il y a 25 pays producteurs, parmi lesquels sept gros producteurs. La production mondiale annuelle d'amiante a culminé vers le milieu des années 70 avec plus de 5 millions de tonnes, mais depuis lors elle a reculé à environ 3 millions de tonnes. Plus de 100 pays fabriquent des produits à base de chrysotile et le Japon en est le principal consommateur. Les grands types d'activités qui sont actuellement susceptibles de provoquer une exposition au chrysotile sont a) l'extraction minière et l'élaboration du matériau (broyage, battage, cardage et filage); b) la fabrication de produits à base de chrysotile (matériaux résistants à la friction, tuyaux et plaques ou feuilles de fibro-ciment, joints, papier, textiles; c) le BTP (construction, réparation et démolition); d) le transport et l'élimination. L'industrie du fibro-ciment ou amiante-ciment est de loin le plus gros utilisateur de fibres de chrysotile puisqu'elle consomme environ 85% de la production.

Lors de la fabrication, de la pose et de l'élimination des produits contenant de l'amiante, de même parfois qu'à l'occasion de l'usure normale de ces produits, il y a libération de fibres. La manipulation de produits friables peut également être une source importante de fibres de chrysotile.

1.3 Concentration sur les lieux de travail et dans l'environnement

D'après des données provenant essentiellement d'Amérique du Nord, d'Europe et du Japon, l'exposition était très importante sur les lieux de travail de la plupart des secteurs de production au cours des années 30.Elle a beaucoup reculé à la fin des années 70 pour descendre finalement aux valeurs actuelles. Au Québec, la concentration atmosphérique moyenne en fibres dans les industries d'extraction et de production a souvent dépassé 20 fibres /ml (f/ml) au cours des années 70, alors qu'elle se situe maintenant en général bien au-dessous de 1 f/ml. Vers la même époque, la concentration moyenne dans l'industrie japonaise du fibro-ciment se caractérisait par des valeurs de l'ordre de 2,5 à 9,5 f/ml, valeurs qui sont tombées à 0,05–0,45 en moyenne en 1992. Dans l'industrie des textiles d'amiante au Japon, la concentration moyenne a été de 2,6 à 12,8 f/ml entre 1970 et 1975, pour reculer à 0,1–0,2 f/ml entre 1984 et 1986.On a observé des tendances analogues dans l'industrie des matériaux antifriction: selon les données provenant de ce même pays, la concentration moyenne a été de 10–35 f/ml entre 1970 et 1975, et de 0,2–5,5 f/ml entre 1984 et 1986. Dans une usine du Royaume-Uni où une vaste étude de mortalité a été effectuée, on mesuré des concentrations généralement supérieures à 20 f/ml avant 1931 et des valeurs généralement inférieures à 1 f/ml pendant la période 1970–1979.

On possède peu de données concernant la concentration en fibres sur les lieux où l'on installe et utilise des produits contenant du chrysotile, bien que ce soit là que les travailleurs ont le plus de chances d'être exposés. Dans des ateliers d'entretien de véhicules, on a enregistré dans les années 70 des pics de concentration atteignant 16 f/ml, alors que depuis 1987, on n'a pratiquement plus jamais mesuré que des valeurs inférieures à 0,2 f/ml. Au cours des années 80, l'exposition moyenne pondérée par rapport au temps lors de la réparation de voitures automobiles a été en général inférieure à 0,05 f/ml. Cependant, faute de contrôle, les débris, en s'envolant des fûts, on fini par donner naissance en peu de temps à de fortes concentrations de poussières.

Résumé

Le personnel chargé de l'entretien court un risque d'exposition à divers types de fibres d'amiante, du fait de la présence de grandes quantités de matériaux asbestiques friables. Dans les bâtiments où une surveillance a été instituée, comme par exemple aux Etats-Unis, l'exposition du personnel d'entretien, exprimée en moyenne pondérée par rapport au temps sur 8 h, se situe entre 0,002 et 0,02 f/ml. Ces valeurs sont du même ordre de grandeur que celles relevées lors de travaux effectués dans des installations de commutation (0, 009 f/ml) ou dans les combles (0,037 f/ml),mais des valeurs plus élevées ont été enregistrées lors de travaux effectués par les services publics (0,5 f/ml). En l'absence de surveillance, la concentration peut être beaucoup plus élevée. Ainsi, dans un cas on a relevé une valeur de 1,6 f/ml lors du balayage d'une pièce et de 15,5 f/ml lors de l'époussetage des livres d'une bibliothèque dans un bâtiment dont les surfaces étaient recouvertes d'un matériau très friable à base de chrysotile. La plupart des autres moyennes pondérées sur 8 h sont d'environ deux ordres de grandeur plus faibles.

Des enquêtes menées avant 1986 ont montré que la teneur en fibres (fibres de plus de 5 µm de longueur) dans l'air extérieur, mesurée en Afrique du Sud, en Allemagne, en Autriche, au Canada et aux Etats-Unis, allait de 0,0001 à 0,001 f/ml environ, la plupart des échantillons contenant moins de 0,01 f/ml. La moyenne ou la médiane s'est située entre 0,00005 et 0,02 f/ml lors de mesures effectuées plus récemment au Canada, aux Etats-Unis, en Italie, au Japon, au Royaume-Uni, en Slovaquie et en Suisse.,

Dans les bâtiments publics, même ceux qui contiennent des matériaux friables à base d'amiante, la concentration des fibres reste dans les limites de celles que l'on mesure dans l'air ambiant. En Allemagne et au Canada, la concentration en fibres (fibres de plus de 5 µm de longueur) relevée avant 1986 dans les immeubles, était généralement inférieure à 0,002 f/ml. Lors d'enquêtes menées plus récemment en Belgique, au Canada, aux Etats-Unis, au Royaume-Uni et en Slovaquie, on a obtenu des valeurs moyennes comprises entre 0,00005 et 0, 0045 f/ml. Seulement 0,67% des fibres de chrysotile avaient plus de 5 µm de longueur).

1.4 Absorption, élimination, rétention et translocation

Après avoir été inhalées, les fibres de chrysotile vont se déposer selon divers paramètres: diamètre aérodynamique, longueur et morphologie. On considère que la plupart des fibres de chrysotile sont respirables du fait que leur diamètre est inférieur à 3 µm, ce qui correspond à un diamètre aérodynamique de 10 µm environ. Chez le rat de laboratoire, les fibres de chrysotile se déposent principalement au niveau de la bifurcation des canaux alvéolaires.

Dans le rhinopharynx et la région trachéobronchique, l'élimination des fibres de chrysotile est assurée par l'ascenseur mucociliaire. Au niveau de la bifurcation des canaux alvéolaires, les fibres sont captées par les cellules épithéliales. L'élimination alvéolaire est conditionnée en grande partie par la longueur des fibres. On est largement fondé à penser, d'après les études sur l'animal, que les fibres courtes (moins de 5 µm de longueur) sont plus rapidement éliminées que les fibres longues (plus de 5 µm de longueur). On ne s'explique pas encore totalement pourquoi les fibres de chrysotile sont éliminées plus rapidement que celles d'amphibole. On a avancé l'hypothèse que les fibres courtes de chrysotile sont phagocytées par les macrophages alvéolaires, les fibres longues étant principalement éliminées par rupture, dissolution ou les deux à la fois. On ne sait pas encore très bien dans quelle proportion les fibres de chrysotile subissent une translocation vers le tissu interstitiel, pleural ou d'autres tissus extrathoraciques.

L'analyse des tissus pulmonaires d'ouvriers exposés à du chrysotile montre que dans le cas de la trémolite, une variété d'amphibole communément présente en petite quantité dans le chrysotile du commerce, la rétention est beaucoup plus importante. L'hypothèse d'une élimination plus rapide du chrysotile est corroborée par l'expérimentation animale, qui montre que cette variété d'amiante est plus vite éliminée des poumons que les amphiboles et notamment la crocidolite et l'amosite.

Les données fournies par les études sur l'homme et l'animal sont insuffisantes pour que l'on puisse déterminer si, et selon quelles modalités, les fibres de chrysotile ingérées sont susceptibles de se fixer, de se répartir dans l'organisme et d'être excrétées. Autant qu'on sache, s'il y a pénétration des fibres de chrysotile à travers la paroi intestinale, elle doit être extrêmement limitée. Selon une étude, il y aurait augmentation du nombre de fibres de chrysotile dans les urines des ouvriers professionnellement exposés à cette variété d'amiante.

1.5 Effets sur les animaux et sur les cellules

De nombreuses études au cours desquelles on a fait inhaler pendant de longues périodes divers échantillons de chrysotile à des rats, ont montré que ces fibres avaient des effets fibrogènes et cancérogènes. Il s'agissait notamment de fibrose interstitielle et de cancers du poumon et de la plèvre. Dans la plupart des cas, on a constaté l'existence d'une association entre la fibrose et les tumeurs pulmonaires chez le rat. Des effets fibrogènes et cancérogènes ont été également mis en évidence lors d'études à long terme sur l'animal (principalement des rats) au cours desquelles on a utilisé d'autres modes d'administration (instillation intratrachéenne et injection intrapleurale ou intrapéritonéale).

Au cours de ces expériences d'inhalation, on n'a pas étudié de manière satisfaisante les relations exposition/dose-réponse dans le cas des fibroses, des cancers pulmonaires et des mésothéliomes induits par le chrysotile. Les études effectuées jusqu'ici, qui ont porté dans la plupart des cas sur une seule concentration, mettent en évidence des effets fibrogènes et cancérogènes à des concentrations en fibres aéroportées allant de 100 à quelques milliers de fibres par ml.

Lorsqu'on regroupe les résultats des différentes études, on voit apparaître une relation entre la concentration atmosphérique des fibres et l'incidence du cancer du poumon. Toutefois, ce genre d'analyse n'est peut-être pas valable sur le plan scientifique, car les conditions expérimentales n'étaient pas identiques dans toutes les études.

Les études qui n'utilisaient pas la voie respiratoire (injection intrapleurale ou intrapéritonéale) ont mis en évidence des relations dose-réponse entre la présence de fibres de chrysotile et l'apparition de mésothéliomes. Cependant, il n'est pas certain que les données obtenues soient utilisable pour évaluer le risque encouru par l'homme en cas d'exposition aux fibres de chrysotile.

La trémolite, qui est un constituant mineur du chrysotile du commerce, s'est également révélée cancérogène et fibrogène chez le rat lors d'une étude comportant une seule inhalation et lors d'une autre étude utilisant la voie intrapéritonéale. On ne dispose pas des données exposition/ dose-réponse qui auraient permis une comparaison directe du pouvoir cancérogène de la trémolite et du chrysotile.

L'aptitude des fibres de chrysotile à provoquer des effets cancérogènes et fibrogènes est fonction de leurs caractéristiques individuelles, notamment les dimensions et la durabilité (c'est-à-dire la biopersistance de la fibre dans les tissus cibles), qui, elle, dépend pour une part des propriétés physico-chimiques de la fibre. L'expérience a amplement montré que les fibres courtes (moins de 5 µm) sont moins actives sur le plan biologique que les longues fibres (plus de 5 µm). Toutefois on ignore encore si les fibres courtes ont la moindre activité biologique. En outre, on ne sait pas combien de temps une fibre doit séjourner dans les poumons pour induire des effets précancéreux, étant donné que l'apparition des cancers liés à l'amiante se produit généralement assez tard dans la vie de l'animal.

Les mécanismes par lesquels le chrysotile et autres matériaux fibreux produisent des effets fibrogènes et cancérogènes ne sont pas totalement élucidés. Dans le cas des effets fibrogènes, il y a peut-être un processus inflammatoire chronique dû à la production de facteurs de croissance (par ex. le TNF-alpha) et d'espèces oxygénées réactives. Dans celui des effets cancérogènes, plusieurs hypothèses ont été avancées. Par exemple: lésion de l'ADN par des espèces oxygénées réactives suscitées par les fibres; lésion directe de l'ADN par suite d'interactions physiques entre les fibres et les cellules cibles; stimulation de la prolifération cellulaire par les fibres; réactions inflammatoires chroniques provoquées par les fibres et conduisant à la libération prolongée d'enzymes lysosomiennes, d'espèces oxygénées réactives, de cytokines et de facteurs de croissance; enfin, action des fibres en tant que co-cancérogènes ou vecteurs de cancérogènes chimiques vers les tissus cibles. En fait, il est probable que tous ces mécanismes interviennent à des degrés divers dans l'activité

Résumé

cancérogène des fibres de chrysotile, car ils ont effectivement été observés *in vitro* dans des systèmes cellulaires humains et mammaliens.

Au total, les données toxicologiques disponibles montrent clairement que les fibres de chrysotile présentent un risque pour l'homme du fait de leur activité fibrogène et cancérogène. Elles ne sont toutefois pas suffisantes pour que l'on puisse en tirer une évaluation quantitative de ce risque. Cela tient au fait que les études utilisant la voie respiratoire n'ont pas fourni de données exposition-réponse suffisantes et aussi aux incertitudes quant à la sensibilité des études sur l'animal pour la prévision du risque chez l'homme.

Plusieurs études de cancérogénicité utilisant la voie buccale ont été consacrées aux fibres de chrysotile. Celles dont on possède les résultats n'ont pas mis en évidence d'effets cancérogènes.

1.6 Effets sur l'homme

Selon de nombreuses études épidémiologiques effectuées sur des travailleurs exposés, l'exposition au chrysotile du commerce accroît le risque de pneumoconiose, de cancer du poumon et de mésothéliome.

Au nombre des affections non malignes attribuables à une exposition au chrysotile, figure tout un ensemble complexe de syndromes cliniques et pathologiques qui ne sont pas suffisamment définis pour que l'on puisse en faire l'étude épidémiologique. On peut citer en premier lieu l'asbestose qui consiste généralement en une fibrose pulmonaire interstitielle diffuse avec une atteinte pleurale plus ou moins importante.

Les études portant sur des travailleurs exposés au chrysotile dans diverses circonstances ont, d'une façon générale, mis en évidence l'existence de relations exposition-réponse et exposition-effet dans le cas de l'asbestose provoquée par le chrysotile, dans la mesure où elles ont permis de constater qu'à un accroissement de l'exposition correspondait une augmentation de l'incidence et de la gravité de la maladie. Il reste toutefois difficile de définir ces relations, en raison de facteurs tels que les incertitudes du diagnostic et la possibilité d'une progression de la maladie après cessation de l'exposition.

En outre, on constate à l'évidence des variations dans l'estimation du risque selon les différentes études. Les raisons de ses variations ne sont pas parfaitement claires, mais il est possible qu'elles tiennent à des incertitudes quant à l'évaluation de l'exposition, à la distribution par taille des fibres atmosphériques selon les diverses industries et aux modèles statistiques utilisés. Il est fréquent d'observer des effets de type asbestosique après une exposition prolongée à des teneurs en fibres de 5 à 20 f/ml.

Les études consacrées aux travailleurs de l'industrie du fibrociment ne font généralement pas état d'un risque relatif élevé de cancer du poumon, ni globalement, ni dans certaines cohortes de travailleurs. La relation exposition-réponse entre le chrysotile et le cancer du poumon correspond à une corrélation 10 à 30 fois plus forte chez les ouvriers du textile que chez ceux des industries d'extraction et de transformation. Le risque relatif de cancer du poumon dans le cas d'expositions cumulées est donc 10 à 30 fois plus élevé chez les ouvriers du textile que chez les mineurs de chrysotile. Les raisons de ces différences demeurent obscures et plusieurs hypothèses ont été avancées pour tenter de les expliquer, notamment des variations dans la distribution de la taille des fibres.

Les études épidémiologiques qui s'efforcent d'évaluer le risque de mésothéliome se heurtent à des difficultés qui tiennent à la rareté de la maladie, à l'absence de statistiques de mortalité pour les populations utilisées comme référence et à un certain nombre de problèmes de diagnostic et de notification. C'est pourquoi, bien souvent, le risque n'est pas calculé et on se contente d'indicateurs plus grossiers, par exemple le nombre absolu de cas et de décès et le rapport du nombre de mésothéliomes au nombre de cancers du poumon ou au nombre total de décès.

Si l'on se base sur les données examinées dans la présente monographie, c'est dans les industries d'extraction et de transformation du chrysotile que le nombre de mésothéliomes est le plus élevé. Chez la totalité des 38 cas observés, il y avait atteinte pleurale,

Résumé

à l'exception d'un seul, entaché d'incertitude, où l'atteinte était pleuro-péritonéale. Aucun mésothéliome n'a été observé chez les travailleurs exposés moins de 2 ans. On a pu dégager une nette relation dose-réponse, avec des taux bruts de mésothéliomes (nombre de cas pour 1000 années-travailleurs) allant de 0,15 pour ceux dont l'exposition cumulée était inférieure à 3530 millions de particules par m^3-années, à 0,97 pour ceux dont l'exposition était supérieure à 10 590 millions de particules par m^3-années.

La proportion de décès attribuables à des mésothéliomes que l'on peut tirer des études de cohortes portant sur les industries d'extraction et de transformation varie de 0 à 0,8%. Il convient d'interpréter ces chiffres avec prudence car les études en question ne fournissent pas des données comparables, avec stratification des décès en fonction de l'intensité et de la durée de l'exposition ainsi que du temps écoulé depuis la première exposition.

On possède un certain nombre d'indices qui donnent à penser que les fibres de trémolite sont à l'origine de mésothéliomes chez l'homme. Comme le chrysotile du commerce est susceptible de contenir de la trémolite fibreuse, on suppose que c'est ce minéral qui provoque l'apparition de mésothéliomes dans certaines populations exposées au chrysotile. On ignore cependant quelle est la relation entre l'excès de mésothéliomes observé et la teneur du chrysotile en trémolite fibreuse.

Les données épidémiologiques ne permettent pas de conclure qu'il y ait une association entre l'exposition au chrysotile et un accroissement du risque de cancers d'autres localisations que la poumon ou la plèvre. Sur ce point, on ne dispose que peu de données au sujet du chrysotile en tant que tel, même si l'on possède quelques indices disparates d'une association entre l'exposition à l'amiante (sous toutes ses formes) et des cancers du larynx, du rein et des voies digestives. Une étude effectuée au Québec sur des mineurs de chrysotile et des ouvriers travaillant à sa transformation, a permis d'observer un excès statistiquement significatif de cancers de l'estomac, mais il est vrai que l'on n'a pas pris en compte la possibilité d'une confusion due au régime alimentaire, aux maladies infectieuses et à d'autres facteurs de risque.

Il faut admettre que, si les études épidémiologiques relatives aux travailleurs exposés au chrysotile se sont cantonnées, pour l'essentiel, aux industries d'extraction et de transformation, il y a lieu de croire, d'après l'histoire naturelle de la maladie et son association à divers types de fibres dans les pays occidentaux, que le risque est probablement plus élevé chez les ouvriers du bâtiment que chez les travailleurs des autres industries.

1.7 Destinée dans l'environnement et effets sur les biotes

Il y a des affleurements de serpentine partout dans le monde. Le travail de l'écorce terrestre provoque l'érosion de ses constituants minéraux et du chrysotile en particulier. Ceux-ci sont transportés à distance et entrent dans le cycle de l'eau, le processus de sédimentation et le profil pédologique. On a trouvé du chrysotile dans l'eau, l'air et dans constituants de l'écorce terrestre et on en a mesuré la teneur.

Le chrysotile et les autres constituants de la serpentine qui lui sont associés subissent une décomposition chimique en surface. Il s'ensuit une modification profonde du pH du sol et l'apparition de traces métalliques dans l'environnement. Toutes ces transformations exercent des effets mesurables sur la croissance des végétaux et des organismes terricoles (notamment les microbes et les insectes), des poissons et des invertébrés. D'après certaines données, des herbivores comme les ovins et les bovins qui ingèrent des graminées poussant sur des sols où affleure la serpentine présentent des modifications de leurs constantes hémochimiques.

1. RESUMEN

1.1 Identidad, propiedades físicas y químicas, muestreo y análisis

El crisotilo es un mineral de silicato de magnesio hidratado fibroso que se ha utilizado en numerosos productos comerciales. En la actualidad se usa ampliamente en el comercio mundial. Se ha observado que sus propiedades físicas y químicas como mineral varían entre los depósitos geológicos explotados. Los minerales que acompañan a las fibras en las menas son muchos y entre ellos puede haber algunas variedades de anfíbol fibroso. Se considera que la tremolita es particularmente importante a este respecto; su forma y concentración presentan grandes variaciones.

En el análisis del crisotilo en los lugares de trabajo se requiere ahora el uso de microscopios ópticos y electrónicos. Antes se habían utilizado diversos instrumentos y dispositivos para vigilar la presencia y concentración tanto de polvo total como de fibras en los diversos medios. En la actualidad se suelen utilizar la técnica del filtro de membrana y la microscopía óptica de contraste de fases para la valoración en el lugar de trabajo (expresada como fibras por ml de aire), y también se emplea la microscopia electrónica de transmisión. Para las valoraciones en el medio ambiente se requiere el uso de la microscopia electrónica de transmisión. Se ha recurrido a estudios de concentración en tejidos para mejorar la información relativa a la exposición. En función del grado de atención al detalle en estos estudios se ha llegado a distintas conclusiones acerca de los mecanismos y la etiología.

Antes se utilizaban las técnicas del precipitador gravimétrico y térmico y el sacudidor de muestreo de polvo para la caracterización en el lugar de trabajo, siendo los valores del polvo (no de la fibra) los únicos índices de exposición inicial para calibrar las relaciones exposición/respuesta. Se ha intentado muchas veces convertir estos valores en los correspondientes a fibras por volumen de aire, pero tales conversiones han tenido un éxito muy limitado. Se ha comprobado que los factores de conversión son específicos de cada industria, e incluso de cada operación; en los factores de conversión universal se han registrado grandes variaciones.

1.2 Fuentes de exposición profesional y ambiental

En todo el medio ambiente de la corteza terrestre (aire, agua, casquetes polares y suelo) se encuentran concentraciones bajas de crisotilo. Las actividades tanto naturales como humanas contribuyen a la aerosolización y la distribución de las fibras. Entre las fuentes de origen humano está el polvo procedente de actividades profesionales, que comprenden la recuperación y elaboración de minerales, la fabricación, la aplicación, la utilización y en último término la eliminación.

Hay producción en 25 países y son siete los principales productores. La producción anual de amianto alcanzó un máximo de más de cinco millones de toneladas a mediados de los años setenta, pero luego ha disminuido hasta el nivel actual de unos tres millones de toneladas. Se fabrican productos de crisotilo en más de 100 países, siendo el Japón el principal consumidor. Las principales actividades actuales de las que se deriva una exposición potencial al crisotilo son las siguientes: a) extracción y trituración; b) transformación en productos (materiales de fricción, tuberías y placas de cemento, juntas y cierres, papel y textiles); c) construcción, reparación y demolición; d) transporte y eliminación. La industria del amianto-cemento es con diferencia la principal usuaria de fibras de crisotilo, absorbiendo alrededor del 85% del total.

Se desprenden fibras durante la elaboración, la instalación y la eliminación de productos con amianto, así como por el desgaste de los productos en algunos casos. La manipulación de productos friables puede ser una fuente importante de emisión de crisotilo.

1.3 Niveles de exposición profesional y ambiental

De acuerdo con datos procedentes sobre todo de América del Norte, de Europa y del Japón, la exposición en los lugares de trabajo a comienzos de los años treinta era muy alta en la mayoría de los sectores de la producción. Los niveles descendieron considerablemente a finales de los años setenta y se ha reducido enormemente hasta los valores actuales. En la industria de la extracción y la trituración de Quebec, las concentraciones medias de fibras en el aire superaban a menudo las 20 fibras/ml (f/ml) en los setenta, mientras que ahora suelen estar muy por debajo de 1 f/ml. En la producción de fibrocemento en el Japón, las concentraciones medias habituales eran de 2,5–9,5 f/ml en los setenta, mientras que en 1992 se notificaron unas concentraciones medias de 0,05–0,45 f/ml. En la fabricación de textiles de amianto en el Japón, las concentraciones medias eran de 2,6 a 12,8 f/ml en el período comprendido entre 1970 y 1975, y de 0,1 a 0,2 f/ml en el período comprendido entre 1984 y 1986. Las tendencias han sido análogas en la producción de materiales de fricción: según los datos disponibles del mismo país, en el período comprendido entre 1970 y 1975 se midieron concentraciones medias de 10–35 f/ml, mientras que entre 1984 y 1986 se notificaron mediciones de 0,2–5,5 f/ml. En una instalación del Reino Unido en la que se realizó un estudio amplio de la mortalidad, las concentraciones eran en general superiores a 20 f/ml en el período anterior a 1931 y normalmente inferiores a 1 f/ml durante 1970–79.

Se dispone de pocos datos sobre las concentraciones de fibras asociadas a la instalación y utilización de productos con crisotilo, aunque fácilmente éste es el lugar de trabajo más probable de exposición de los trabajadores. En el mantenimiento de los vehículos se notificaban en los años setenta concentraciones máximas de hasta 16 f/ml, mientras que prácticamente todos los niveles medidos después de 1987 fueron de menos de 0,2 f/ml. Las exposiciones medias ponderadas por el tiempo durante la reparación de vehículos de pasajeros en los años ochenta eran por lo general inferiores a 0,05 f/ml. Sin embargo, en ausencia de controles la descarga de residuos de los cilindros daba lugar a concentraciones elevadas de polvo de corta duración.

Existe la posibilidad de exposición de personal de mantenimiento a diversos tipos de fibras de amianto debido a la elevada cantidad de amianto friable en su lugar de trabajo. En edificios con planes de control de los Estados Unidos, la exposición del personal de mantenimiento de edificios expresada como promedio ponderado por el tiempo durante ocho horas fue de 0,002 a 0,02 f/ml. Estos valores son del mismo orden de magnitud que las exposiciones normales durante el trabajo de los operadores de telecomunicaciones (0,009 f/ml) y al aire libre (0,037 f/ml), aunque se notificaron concentraciones mayores en lugares de trabajo de espacios cerrados (0,5 f/ml). Las concentraciones pueden ser considerablemente más elevadas cuando no se han introducido planes de control. En un caso se detectaron concentraciones episódicas de corta duración de 1,6 f/ml al barrer y de 15,5 f/ml mientras se limpiaba el polvo de los libros de una biblioteca en un edificio con un tipo de superficie que contenía crisotilo muy friable. La mayoría de los demás promedios ponderados por el tiempo durante ocho horas son alrededor de dos órdenes de magnitud menores.

De acuerdo con los estudios realizados antes de 1986, las concentraciones de fibras (fibras > 5 µ de longitud) en el aire exterior, medidas en Alemania, Austria, el Canadá, los Estados Unidos y Sudáfrica, oscilaban entre 0,0001 y alrededor de 0,01 f/ml, siendo los niveles de la mayoría de las muestras menores de 0,001 f/ml. Las medias o las medianas eran de 0,00005 a 0,02 f/ml, tomando como base determinaciones más recientes en el Canadá, los Estados Unidos, Italia, el Japón, el Reino Unido, la República Eslovaca y Suiza.

Las concentraciones de fibras en edificios públicos, incluso los que tienen materiales con amianto friable, son del orden de las medidas en el aire exterior. Las concentraciones (fibras > 5 µ de longitud) en edificios de Alemania y el Canadá notificadas antes de 1986 eran en general menores de 0,002 f/ml. En estudios más recientes realizados en Bélgica, el Canadá, los Estados Unidos, el Reino Unido y la República Eslovaca se obtuvieron valores medios de 0,00005 a 0,0045 f/ml. Sólo un 0,67% de las fibras de crisotilo eran más largas de 5 µ.

1.4 Absorción, eliminación, retención y desplazamiento

La deposición del crisotilo inhalado depende del diámetro aerodinámico, la longitud y la morfología de la fibra. La mayoría de las fibras de crisotilo transportadas por el viento se consideran respirables debido a que su diámetro es de menos de 3 µ, igual a un diámetro aerodinámico de 10 µ. En ratas de laboratorio, las fibras de crisotilo se depositan principalmente en las bifurcaciones de los conductos alveolares.

En las regiones nasofaríngea y traqueobronquial, las fibras de crisotilo se eliminan por medio de la acción mucociliar. Las células epiteliales absorben las fibras en las bifurcaciones de los conductos alveolares. La longitud de las fibras es un factor determinante importante para la eliminación alveolar de las fibras de crisotilo. Hay pruebas convincentes obtenidas en estudios con animales de que las fibras cortas (de menos de 5 µ de longitud) se eliminan con mayor rapidez que las largas (de más de 5 µ). No se conocen completamente los mecanismos que hacen que las fibras de crisotilo se eliminen de manera relativamente más rápida que las de anfíboles. Se ha planteado la hipótesis de que las fibras cortas de crisotilo pueden eliminarse sobre todo por fagocitosis de los macrófagos alveolares, mientras que las largas lo harían principalmente por rotura y/o disolución. No se conoce del todo en qué medida se desplazan las fibras de crisotilo a los intersticios, al tejido pleural y a otros tejidos extratorácicos.

Los análisis de los pulmones de trabajadores expuestos al crisotilo ponen de manifiesto una retención de tremolita, amianto anfíbol que suele estar asociado con el crisotilo comercial en pequeñas proporciones, mucho mayor que la de crisotilo. La eliminación más rápida de las fibras de crisotilo de los pulmones humanos se ha confirmado en los resultados de estudios con animales, que mostraban que el crisotilo se elimina de los pulmones con mayor rapidez que los anfíboles, incluidas la crocidolita y la amosita.

Los datos obtenidos en estudios con personas y con animales son insuficientes para evaluar la posible absorción, distribución y excreción de fibras de crisotilo a partir de la ingestión. Las pruebas disponibles indican que, en el caso de que se produzca penetración de fibras de crisotilo a través de las paredes del intestino, es extraordinariamente limitada. En un estudio se observó una concentración mayor de fibras de crisotilo en la orina de trabajadores expuestos profesionalmente al crisotilo.

1.5 Efectos en animales y en células

En numerosos estudios de inhalación de larga duración se ha comprobado que diversas muestras experimentales de fibras de crisotilo provocan efectos fibrogénicos y carcinogénicos en ratas de laboratorio. Entre esos efectos figuran la fibrosis intersticial y el cáncer de pulmón y de pleura. En la mayoría de los casos parece haber una asociación entre fibrosis y tumores en el pulmón de rata. También se han detectado efectos fibrogénicos y carcinogénicos en estudios de larga duración con animales (principalmente ratas) utilizando otras vías de administración (por ejemplo, instilación intratraqueal e inyección intrapleural o intraperitoneal).

No se han investigado debidamente en estudios de inhalación de larga duración en animales las relaciones exposición/dosis-respuesta para la fibrosis pulmonar, el cáncer de pulmón y el mesotelioma inducidos por el crisotilo. Los estudios de inhalación realizados hasta la fecha, utilizando sobre todo una concentración de exposición única, muestran respuestas fibrogénicas y carcinogénicas a concentraciones de fibras en el aire que van de 100 a algunos miles de fibras/ml. Al combinar los datos de varios estudios, parece que hay una relación entre las concentraciones de fibras en el aire y la incidencia de cáncer de pulmón. Sin embargo, este tipo de análisis tal vez no sea válido desde el punto de vista científico, debido a que las condiciones experimentales en los estudios disponibles eran distintas.

En los experimentos sin inhalación (estudios de inyección intrapleural e intraperitoneal), se ha demostrado una relación dosis-respuesta para el mesotelioma con las fibras de crisotilo. Sin embargo, es posible que los datos de estos estudios no sean adecuados para evaluar el riesgo humano derivado de la exposición a fibras por inhalación.

El amianto tremolita, mineral que es un componente secundario del crisotilo comercial, también mostró efectos carcinogénicos y fibrogénicos en un experimento de inhalación única y en un estudio de inyección intraperitoneal en ratas. No se dispone de datos sobre la exposición/dosis respuesta para poder establecer una comparación directa de la actividad carcinogénica de la tremolita y el crisotilo.

Resumen

La capacidad de las fibras para inducir efectos fibrogénicos y carcinogénicos parece depender de sus características individuales, incluidas la dimensión y la durabilidad de las fibras (es decir, la biopersistencia en los tejidos a los que llegan), que están determinadas en parte por las propiedades fisicoquímicas. Está bien documentado en estudios experimentales el hecho de que las fibras cortas (de menos de 5 μ) tienen una actividad biológica menor que las largas (de más de 5 μ). Sin embargo, sigue habiendo dudas acerca de si las fibras cortas tienen una actividad biológica significativa. Además, no se sabe cuánto tiempo tiene que permanecer una fibra en el pulmón para inducir efectos preneoplásicos, puesto que el cáncer relacionado con el amianto suele aparecer en una etapa posterior de la vida del animal.

No se conocen completamente los mecanismos mediante los cuales el crisotilo y otras fibras provocan efectos fibrogénicos y carcinogénicos. Entre los posible mecanismos de los efectos fibrogénicos de las fibras cabe mencionar el proceso de inflamación crónica debido a la producción de factores del crecimiento (por ejemplo, el TNF-alfa) y especies de oxígeno reactivo. Con respecto a la carcinogenicidad inducida por las fibras, se han propuesto varias hipótesis. Son las siguientes: daños en el ADN provocados por especies de oxígeno reactivo inducido por las fibras; daños directos en el ADN por las interacciones físicas entre las fibras y las células a las que llegan; intensificación de la proliferación celular debida a las fibras; reacciones inflamatorias crónicas provocadas por las fibras, que da lugar a una liberación prolongada de lisozimas, especies reactivas de oxígeno, citoquinas y factores del crecimiento; y actuación de las fibras como agentes cocarcinógenos o portadores de productos químicos carcinógenos hasta los tejidos a los que llegan. Es probable, sin embargo, que todos estos mecanismos contribuyan a la carcinogenicidad de las fibras de crisotilo, puesto que se han observado tales efectos en diversos sistemas *in vitro* de células humanas y de mamíferos.

En conjunto, los datos toxicológicos disponibles demuestran claramente que las fibras de crisotilo pueden crear peligros fibrogénicos y carcinogénicos para el ser humano. Sin embargo, los datos no son suficientes para obtener estimaciones cuantitativas del riesgo para las personas. Esto se debe a que son insuficientes los procedentes de estudios de inhalación relativos a la exposición-respuesta y a que hay dudas cerca de la sensibilidad de los estudios con animales para predecir el riesgo humano.

Se han realizado pruebas con fibras de crisotilo en varios estudios de carcinogenicidad por vía oral. En los estudios disponibles no se han notificado efectos carcinogénicos.

1.6 Efectos en el ser humano

Las calidades comerciales de crisotilo se han asociado con un aumento del riesgo de neumoconiosis, cáncer de pulmón y mesotelioma en numerosos estudios epidemiológicos de trabajadores expuestos.

Las enfermedades no malignas asociadas con la exposición al crisotilo forman una mezcla algo compleja de síndromes clínicos y patológicos imposibles de definir para un estudio epidemiológico. La preocupación se ha concentrado primordialmente en la asbestosis, que generalmente consiste en una enfermedad asociada con una fibrosis pulmonar intersticial difusa acompañada de diversos grados de afección pleural.

Los estudios realizados en trabajadores expuestos al crisotilo en distintos sectores han demostrado en general una relación exposición-respuesta o exposición-efecto para la asbestosis inducida por crisotilo, puesto que el aumento de los niveles de exposición ha producido un incremento de la incidencia y la gravedad de la enfermedad. Sin embargo, hay dificultades para definir esta relación, debido a factores como la incertidumbre del diagnóstico y la posibilidad de progresión de la enfermedad después de cesar la exposición.

Por otra parte, entre los estudios disponibles son evidentes algunas variaciones en las estimaciones del riesgo. Los motivos de estas variaciones no son totalmente claros, pero pueden estar relacionados con la incertidumbre en las estimaciones de la exposición, la distribución por tamaños de las fibras del aire en los diversos sectores industriales y los modelos estadísticos. Son habituales los cambios en la asbestosis tras exposiciones prolongadas a concentraciones de 5 a 20 f/ml.

Los riesgos relativos totales de cáncer de pulmón no son por lo general elevados en los estudios realizados con trabajadores de la producción de fibrocemento y en algunas de las cohortes de trabajadores de fábricas de fibrocemento. La relación exposición-respuesta entre el crisotilo y el riesgo de cáncer de pulmón parece ser en los estudios de trabajadores textiles 10–30 veces mayor que en los estudios de trabajadores de las industrias de la extracción y la trituración. No están claros los motivos de esta variación del riesgo, por lo que se han propuesto varias hipótesis, incluidas las variaciones de la distribución de las fibras por tamaños.

La estimación del riesgo de mesotelioma se complica en los estudios epidemiológicos debido a factores como la rareza de la enfermedad, la falta de tasas de mortalidad en las poblaciones utilizadas como referencia y los problemas de diagnóstico y notificación. Por consiguiente, en muchos casos no se han calculado los riesgos y se han utilizado indicadores más aproximativos, como el número absoluto de casos y de muertes y la razón mesotelioma/cáncer de pulmón o número total de muertes.

Tomando como base los datos reseñados en esta monografía, el mayor número de mesoteliomas se ha registrado en el sector de la extracción y la trituración del crisotilo. Los 38 casos fueron pleurales con la excepción de uno de probabilidad baja de diagnóstico, que fue pleuroperitoneal. No se produjo ningún caso en trabajadores expuestos durante menos de dos años. Se observó una relación dosis-respuesta clara, con tasas brutas de mesoteliomas (casos/1000 años-persona) comprendidas entre 0,15 para los casos de una exposición acumulativa a menos de 3530 millones de partículas/m^3-año (< 1000 millones de partículas por pie cúbico-año) y 0,97 para los de una exposición a más de 10 590 millones de partículas/m^3-año (> 300 millones de partículas/pie cúbico-año).

Las proporciones de muertes atribuibles a mesoteliomas en estudios de cohortes en los diversos sectores de la extracción y la producción oscilan entre el 0% y el 0,8%. Estas proporciones se han de interpretar con cautela, puesto que los estudios no suministran datos comparables con una estratificación de las muertes por intensidades de exposición, duración de ésta o tiempo transcurrido desde la primera.

Hay pruebas de que la tremolita fibrosa provoca la aparición de mesoteliomas en el ser humano. Debido a que el crisotilo comercial puede contener tremolita fibrosa, se ha planteado la hipótesis de que ésta puede contribuir a la inducción de mesoteliomas en algunas poblaciones expuestas primordialmente al crisotilo. No se ha determinado en qué medida podría atribuirse el aumento observado de mesoteliomas al contenido de tremolita fibrosa.

No se han obtenido pruebas epidemiológicas concluyentes de que la exposición al crisotilo esté asociada con un mayor riesgo de tipos de cáncer distintos del de pulmón o el de pleura. Hay información limitada acerca de este tema para el crisotilo en sí, pero no son convincentes las pruebas aducidas para demostrar una asociación entre la exposición al amianto (todas las formas) y el cáncer de laringe, el de riñón y el gastrointestinal. Se ha observado un aumento significativo de cáncer de estómago en un estudio de mineros y trituradores de crisotilo de Quebec, pero no se ha examinado la posible confusión con la alimentación, con la presencia de infecciones y con otros factores de riesgo.

Hay que reconocer que, aunque los estudios epidemiológicos de trabajadores expuestos al crisotilo se han limitado fundamentalmente a la extracción y la trituración, así como al sector de la fabricación, existen pruebas, basadas en la evolución histórica de las enfermedades asociadas con la exposición a mezclas de diversos tipos de fibras en los países occidentales, de que probablemente los riesgos sean mayores entre los trabajadores de la construcción y posiblemente entre los de otras industrias que utilizan el producto.

1.7 Destino en el medio ambiente y efectos en la biota

En todo el mundo hay afloramientos de serpentina. Los componentes minerales, entre ellos el crisotilo, se erosionan como consecuencia de los procesos de la corteza terrestre y se transportan hasta convertirse en un componente del ciclo hídrico, los sedimentos y el perfil del suelo. Se ha medido la presencia y las concentraciones de crisotilo en el agua, el aire y otras unidades de la corteza.

El crisotilo y los minerales de serpentina asociados con él se degradan químicamente en la superficie. Esto da lugar a cambios profundos del pH del suelo e introduce una serie de metales traza en el medio ambiente. Esto ha producido a su vez efectos mensurables en el crecimiento de las plantas, la biota del suelo (incluidos microorganismos e insectos), los peces y los invertebrados. Algunos datos indican que los animales de pastoreo (ovinos y vacunos) sufren cambios de la química sanguínea tras la ingestión de gramíneas que han crecido en afloramientos de serpentina.

www.ingramcontent.com/pod-product-compliance
Ingram Content Group UK Ltd.
Pitfield, Milton Keynes, MK11 3LW, UK
UKHW021312180426
11947UKWH00015B/1190